The 12 Pillars of Vibrant Health

LOOKING GOOD AND FEELING GREAT...
THE ANTI-AGING AND LONGEVITY FORMULA

SCOTT SOMMER LAC

SPOTLIGHT
PUBLISHING HOUSE

Goodyear, Arizona

The 12 Pillars of Vibrant Health
–Looking Good and Feeling Great… The Anti-Aging and Longevity Formula

eBook ISBN: 978-1-962570-82-4
Paperback ISBN: 978-1-962570-83-1
Hardcover ISBN: 978-1-962570-85-5
Ingram Spark ISBN: 978-1-962570-84-8
Library of Congress Control Number: 2024916340

Editor: Carolyn Sommer
Co-Editor: Bethany Good – Good Writing Inc.
Cover Image: Adobe Stock
Cover Design: Angela Alaya
Interior Design: Marigold 2k
Publisher: Spotlight Publishing House –
https://spotlightpublishinghouse.com

Disclaimer: This book is not intended as a substitute for the medical advice of physicians. The reader should regularly consult a physician in matters relating to their health, particularly with respect to any symptoms that may require diagnosis or medical attention. All nutritional guidance and dietary suggestions are for informational purposes only. Individuals with specific dietary needs or health concerns should consult a registered dietician or physician.

Check Out Our Website!
https://www.sommersholistichealth.com

Endorsements

"In today's world of unprecedented challenges to our health, this book is a timely tome of timeless truth about how to thrive, not just survive. My colleague Scott Sommer has done an excellent job of combining hard-won lessons from his own personal health challenges, the ancient wisdom of Chinese medicine, and leading-edge science of mind-body health to give the reader proven and practical steps towards a vibrant life well-lived. Scott artfully blends valuable insights on body, mind and spirit to help lift the reader to a higher level of life, contribution and vitality. I highly recommend this book."

–Dr Michael Gaeta, DAOM, MS
Director, Gaeta Institute for Wholistic Health Education, and the Gaeta Clinic

"Natural healthcare is critically important in life and this book supports people in achieving that. The soil, seed and growing process has changed over the last 50 years, and we all need to change our lifestyles to adapt to the nutrient deficiencies.

READ THIS BOOK and start changing YOUR LIFE and the lives around YOU for the better."

–Charles C. DuBois, President and CEO, Standard Process Inc

"I want to acknowledge Scott Sommer's care and intense research to help people resolve physical issues so they can live optimum and healthy lives. I have known and worked with Scott for over 10 years, witnessing his undying persistence in helping individuals and families.

Thank you, Scott and your team for your dedication. It is truly needed and appreciated."
–**Rohn Walker**, CEO International Executive Technology

"As a friend and colleague of Scott Sommer Lac, I've had the privilege of witnessing firsthand his dedication to holistic health and wellness. *The 12 Pillars of Vibrant Health* is not just a book to me; it's a culmination of Scott's profound knowledge and genuine passion for helping others live their best lives.

In my own journey towards well-being, Scott has been an invaluable resource. He's not just on my shortlist of healthcare professionals; he's often the first person I reach out to when I need a second, and often better, brain than mine. His insights, rooted in traditional Chinese medicine and complemented by modern science, have consistently enriched my understanding of health and empowered me to make positive changes.

Through *The 12 Pillars of Vibrant Health*, Scott shares his wealth of wisdom with readers, offering practical guidance and profound insights to help them achieve holistic vitality. Whether you're looking to improve your diet, enhance your fitness routine, or cultivate mindfulness, Scott's holistic approach provides a roadmap for lasting transformation.

I wholeheartedly endorse *The 12 Pillars of Vibrant Health* to anyone seeking to elevate their health and well-being. Scott's unique blend of expertise, compassion, and dedication shines through every page, inspiring readers to embrace a life of vitality, balance, and joy."
–**Dustin Strong,** CHN-BC, CAN
Holistic Nutritionist | Health, Wellness and Lifestyle Counselor | Educational Speaker, STRONG ON HEALTH

Contents

Dedication and Acknowledgements

I dedicate this book to the many people in my life who have supported, inspired, encouraged, and directed me throughout my life, enabling me to reach this pinnacle in my career.

Most importantly, I would like to acknowledge the Lord and His faithfulness to me throughout my life. He has walked with me on this journey of faith since the beginning.

Through every trial He has directed my steps with unmerited grace, beginning with the healing of my childhood epilepsy. I give Him all the glory for my success as He continues to send patients I can help and a deep love to serve them as well.

After completing many years of education, I asked the Lord in prayer "How will they find me?" He said, "Fear not, I will send them to you, and I will give you wisdom to fully restore their health." He has remained faithful to that promise and remains my ever-present help with each patient. When colleagues ask me where I learned so much, I tell them from the great physician, the Lord.

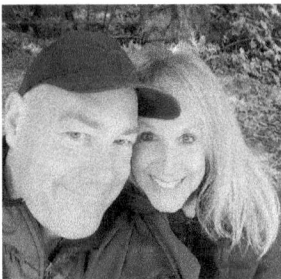

To Carolyn, my wife, my soul mate, and my best friend. My rock star editor. Though we met later in life, I feel we've been together for years. I appreciate your willingness to take on new ideas. Your continued support no matter what comes our way, your tenacity, and inspiration. You are my inspiration. You are a superstar. God blessed me with the best of the best. Love you forever!

To my Dad, who pushed me to my outer limits, and taught me to work hard. He pushed me to do my best no matter how small the project. Working with him as a youth on the farm and on difficult job sites prepared me for life. I learned to plan ahead, as I watched him load the work van, days in advance preparing for a job, making sure he had the best tools for any problem we might face. He always said, "Never waste a stroke

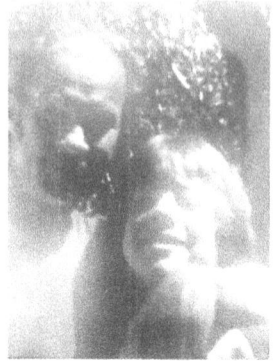

My Dad and Me.

when paper hanging." To this day I never waste a stroke and strive for perfection. He taught me that good food comes from good soil. He said, "The Lord speaks, so shoot beyond what seems possible."

My Mom – She was my biggest fan and biggest cheer leader. She was my joyful example of laughter and hard work. She was a single mom while raising me and insisted I get a good education, without which I would not be where I am today. She sent me to a Lutheran School where I met the Lord, and for that I will be forever grateful. I learned to love, forgive, and accept people where they're at because of her example.

To my kids, for making me a proud papa, Natalia, Shy and Johnny. To all my bonus kids Robert, Steven, Sarah, Susanna and Rachel. Thank you for accepting me late in the game.

To Avery, I am grateful for all your hard work, and so proud of you. Together we created great content in preparation for this book.

To Ken and Verna, I appreciate you both in believing in me over the years. So many Saturdays at your home in Orangevale to bring this book to life.

Mentors in Education

Mr. Carl Eastwood
Who said to me in 7th grade, "You're really going somewhere!" and I believed you.

Mrs. Lang
All of our music lessons together and words of encouragement. Believing in me so I believed in myself. Good music is healing to the soul!

Mentors

Carolyn Reuben
You believed in me.

Judith Levy
Thank you for introducing me to Standard Process, muscle testing, and providing my first room. I will always remember your playful nature. You pushed me to the next level when you told me, "If you don't test it's a guess." Life changing words!

Michael Dobbins
A legend, you made nutrition a comedy skit, so grateful for finding you so early in my career. Thank you!

Brian Tracy
A mentor for many years.

Dr. Ulan
Taught me to read the body like a book by teaching me nutrition response testing.

Dr. Michael Gaeta
For being a great example and leader in our profession.

Dustin Strong
For your encouragement, as iron sharpening iron.

Legends of the Past:

Dr. Royal Lee for his incredible legacy and research.

Jack LaLanne for setting the standard and setting an amazing example.

Publishing Support Team:

Becky Norwood – Spotlight Publishing House
For believing in me and helping me to finish this book. We made it to the finish line.

You have always been so gracious and supportive.

Bethany Good – Co-Editor
I'm so grateful for your help and patience.

Tips and Goals for This Book

1. Start a journal while reading. Write down all the changes you're going to make chapter by chapter. Journaling is an important way for the mind and body to connect, recording the inspirations while reading the chapters. It is what you want to do and what you need to do to make things a habit. When we write things down and commit to them, it is the beginning of greatness, like so many that have come before us and have shown us throughout history.

2. Decide on your life purpose and gifts. What is your purpose and your divine destiny? What are you passionate about? What comes naturally? What talents? Write them down and set goals that align with that divine mission and purpose every day. Then, every week and month, review and reassess to make sure you're heading in the right direction to achieve those goals.

3. Make sure you find a friend to talk to about your new goals. This will change your life tremendously and bring accountability in carrying them out. Just one degree of change each day with food, nutrition, lifestyle, and mindset can change the course of your future self.

4. Make changes slowly. Master one change for 30 days before you add on a new change.

"America is over-fed and under-nourished."
Scott Sommer, LAc

"Stand at the crossroads and look.
Ask for the ancient paths. Ask for where the good way is
and walk in it, and you will find rest for your souls."
Jeremiah 16:5

Preface

"For I know the plans I have for you, declares the Lord,
plans to give you a hope and a future."
—Jeremiah 29:11

Just as the verse above was intended to inspire you and give you hope, the purpose of this book is to inspire each of you to become all you can be and to fulfill your God-given purpose. After 26 years of clinical practice, I have seen lives transformed time and time again.

Many today believe common conditions such as diabetes, heart disease, cancer, auto-immune, obesity, and arthritis are all normal as you age. I see patients everyday with these common conditions and more.

Many children and adults are labeled with hopeless physical or psychological conditions and are told they will permanently have to depend on drugs to manage their lifestyles. I was one of those people. I was diagnosed with epilepsy as a child and told by doctors that I would never have a normal life. Shunned by family members, embarrassed and ashamed, I lived with my diagnosis. Yet, something happened at the age of 9 after I left the doctor's office in despair. I went home and prayed for answers from God. I promised Him that if He would heal my brain, I would dedicate the rest of my life to healing other people's brains. The following quote changed my life…

"Let food be thy medicine, and medicine be thy food."
—Hippocrates

I took that to heart and began my healing journey and was declared free of epilepsy at age 15. I studied the book "Back to Eden," herbal medicine and nutrition, determined to find the answers.

I discovered ancient secrets in the Garden of Eden which have continued to heal the body. Within these pages I intend to share those secrets with you. It is my hope that *The 12 Pillars of Vibrant Health* will inspire and motivate you to make the necessary changes in your own life to achieve the end goal of a vibrant and abundant life.

Since the beginning, men and women have taken things into their own hands, and people have gotten away from the foods and lifestyles that produce life and vibrance in our hearts minds and bodies.

Instead, we choose dead foods, slothful lifestyles, and make careless choices concerning our health. Not intentionally, but after the industrial revolution we embraced fast, cheap, and convenient foods. This has paved the way to the emergency room with dire consequences while putting our hope in pharmaceutical drugs and fast medicine, both of which cover up symptoms and ignore the root cause. Farmers of old knew that nutrition begins with the soil. Yet now, large corporations control the farming industry and farm for profit alone, no longer concerned about the nutritional value. The focus has become – farm fast, cheap, and profitable regardless of the consequences.

"One salad will not change your life, but a 100 will."
Scott Sommer, LAc

Lifestyle is a Choice

I see lives transformed everyday as my patients embrace their challenges, and overcome the generational habits and addictions handed down to them by their parents. You don't have to suffer from diabetes, high blood pressure, or arthritis. You can reverse disease naturally and safely without drugs, by simply embracing your health and fulfilling your purpose.

"You never know how much better you can feel until you feel your best. The best is yet to come with hope, hard work and determination."
Scott Sommer, LAc

Introduction

I was diagnosed with epilepsy at 18 months old. My parents spent much of my childhood submitting to doctors and medication. The medication numbed my brain and made me depressed. When I was just nine years old, my pediatrician told me I would never have a normal life. He didn't tell me why I had epilepsy or what to do about it, so I went home feeling depressed and helpless. Until I went up to my room, looked out the window, stared at a tree and prayed. I knew there had to be a natural way to overcome epilepsy. I asked the Lord to give me the powers of superman with x-ray vision to figure out what it was and what I had to do. I couldn't accept what the doctors were saying. I was determined to overcome it. I had to believe that despite my diagnosis and with God's help I could change my destiny. I made a promise to the Lord that if He would fix my brain, then I would dedicate the rest of my life to fixing other people's brains.

I began reading everything I could on nutrition and disease and found the answers to help me on my journey. I spent hours as a child reading nutrition books and listening to Jack LaLanne, Adele Davis, and the most incredible mentor of all: my dad, an organic farmer and bodybuilder who lived off his land. I began making several lifestyle changes, exercising regularly, eating good fats for the brain, getting more sleep and drinking plenty of water. I learned to think positively and to have a great attitude. Yet through it all I knew my faith in God was my strength and the reason I was healed. When I was 15, I was retested by doctors and after three hours of multiple tests they told me I was free of epilepsy. Yet, they had no idea what caused it or how I managed to overcome it. They just told me to go live my life. So, that's exactly what I did, and am still doing to this day – living my best life, serving the Lord by serving others, and fulfilling my God given destiny.

I knew prayer and determination played a huge part in changing my outlook and ultimately, my life. I have never let anyone's discouraging comments or life's obstacles stop me from achieving my purpose. I attended UC Davis as a pre-med student. I discovered then western medicine does not teach about the root cause of disease. They taught pharmaceuticals and surgery. I knew from my own experience the root cause could be found in food and lifestyle, yet they didn't teach anything about nutrition. This caused doubt in my mind about working as a western medicine doctor. One day I went to the library and found a book on Ancient Oriental medicine. I read it for four hours, discovering the body and every cell was electric. I knew then what direction I wanted to go. So, I changed my major to Nutritional Science, knowing then I wanted to pursue a degree in Oriental medicine. After receiving my bachelor's degree in Nutritional Science from UC Davis, I began pursuing a Master's in Oriental Medicine. I was continually mocked and criticized for this by my own extended family. They laughed at me, scoffed at my goals, and told me I was wasting my time. I had an uncle who said, "Alternative medicine? How will you ever make a living doing that?" No one supported my goals except my parents. Yet, here I am, 26 years later, with a thriving medical practice and thousands of patients behind me. You must have faith, know and believe in yourself, and turn a deaf ear to those who don't believe in you. Success is the greatest satisfaction in the face of adversity.

I wrote *"The 12 Pillars to Vibrant Health,"* to inspire and motivate you to make the necessary changes in your own life. Why are so many sick and dying around us? Young and old are suffering from common ailments and terminal diseases. Surely, this was not the plan for our lives. Yet here we are riddled with disease and devastating outcomes – the secret lies in the beginning with the Garden of Eden.

"Dust off your Bible and embrace the Ancient way of healing."
Scott Sommer, LAc

Scan the QR Code below with your smartphone to view:
Achieve Your Health Goals

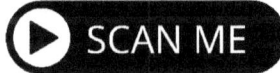

Or follow this link: https://qrco.de/achievehealthgoals

Go to the ant, thou sluggard; consider her ways, and be wise:
Which having no guide, overseer, or ruler, provides her meat
in the summer, and gathers her food in the harvest.
–Proverbs 6:6-8

We can learn a lot from the ants about discipline and diligence. If each of us were as disciplined and diligent about our health, we would have the abundant life that we were intended to have. Every animal, insect, and plant has a divine purpose to fulfill, and so do we. We have a divine purpose to fulfill every day with 8 hours to work, 8 hours to sleep, and 8 hours to enjoy. We have 16 hours to fulfill our purpose. Yet, we cannot fulfill our purpose if we are sick, slothful, and careless about the foods we eat and the lifestyles we live. I have studied the parallels between animals and people. Animals instinctively live the life our creator intended for them to live unless they are sent to a zoo or caged by their owners. When an animal cannot fulfill its divine purpose, it becomes slothful, fat, and tired. It ceases to thrive, it suffers from poor health, and it loses its motivation to do what it was created to do. We are not able to thrive in life and fulfill our purpose if our physical bodies are continually suffering and hindering us.

What We Eat and What We Do Matters

Each day is a new day to make the right choices. I see lives transformed every day as my patients embrace their challenges and overcome the generational habits and addictions handed down to them by their parents. You can reverse disease naturally and safely without drugs by simply embracing your health and deciding to do what you need to to do to be healthy.

In conclusion, I hope you find new hope and inspiration to live a vibrant, joyful, and hope-filled life, regardless of what you have been told by your family, friends, or doctors. You too, can discover the formula of vibrant health and experience the thrill of success as I did at age 15 when I was declared free of epilepsy.

When was the last time you felt great? There's no stopping aging, but you can pump the brakes. You can fight back, feel great, fulfill your God-given destiny, and live the abundant life you were intended to live. I am living proof of that.

"Since the fall of Adam we have been aging. Every day, our bodies break down. The real choice is whether we age gracefully or faster than necessary. Aging gracefully in my mind is like a classic car. It's well taken care of, and it lasts longer than you would ever expect it to, and it looks like an older car in mint condition."
Scott Sommer, LAc

Scan the QR Code below with your
smartphone to view:
SCOTT'S STORY

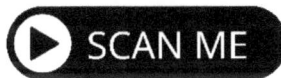

Or follow this link: https://qrco.de/scottsommerstory

Chapter 1

Mindset

"As a Man Thinketh so is he."
—Proverbs 23:7

"Attitude is Altitude." I learned this early in life, and it has been my motto throughout my life. Plan on a great day and great things can happen. The beginning of change always starts with your mindset.

The origin of disease can often be traced back to negative emotions like worry, hopelessness, bitterness, anger, etc. These emotions hinder people from embracing a vibrant life. Just as success can be traced back to a positive self-image, determination, goals, and diligence, our mindset is connected to how we think of ourselves, our emotions, and how we feel about others.

What are you grateful for? When we are grateful, a vibrant life often follows. Our thoughts have a direct effect on our life journey and our health journey. This is the first pillar to vibrant health. Finding something to be grateful for each morning despite our circumstances and doing the things that bring you joy are together the gateway to our own vibrant health and life.

So often, the only voice we hear in our head is our own, especially when it comes to pursuing health. We are often surrounded by friends and family who are not on the same page. So, at the end of the day, our mindset and determination are all we have. You become who you want to be by knowing what you want to be and envisioning yourself as that person. You must believe you can make things happen and overcome challenges, whether it be mentally, physically, spiritually, or emotionally.

It's up to you to decide what you want from your day. This is your mindset. This is how you determine how you will feel on any given day. If you wake up thinking, "This is going to be a bad day," I guarantee it will be, but if you wake up just grateful to be alive and decide it will be a fantastic day, most likely it will be. Remember, Attitude is altitude.

Tip:

Every morning, start your day with a smile even if you don't feel like it, hold it until you feel the smile overcome you and you're ready to start your day!

How to Overcome Obstacles

If you find yourself struggling emotionally and physically remember these principles.

- There is hope and help through every struggle.
- Remember it takes determination and change to overcome every struggle or diagnosis.
- Developing new habits is like climbing a mountain. It always feels great when you get to the top. The view is amazing!

There Are Two Types of People

The first is a cup with a lid on it. Narrow-minded, unwilling to learn anything new, and reluctant to expand their horizons or to embrace new ideas. In effect, it equates to a closed-minded person.

The second is a flowing river. Forever expanding their knowledge, expanding their life, and flowing through life, like a river with no boundaries. With a positive and open mind, helping them to overcome struggles, either physically or emotionally.

You've probably seen the stories of people who have become paralyzed, lost limbs, or have a terminal illness. They choose to embrace it with determination and a positive attitude. It's hard for some of us to imagine this, yet these people defy the odds with unbelievable strength and vigor and often encourage those around them to do the same. They have made a choice to accept what is tragic and turn it into an incredible story of strength and resilience.

Your mindset is the first and most important aspect of overcoming health struggles and obstacles in your path. A negative mindset will keep you stuck and sick. When you reach a pivotal fork in the road, you will either remain stuck in a negative place, deciding there's no point in trying, or embrace it as a mountain to climb. When you have a positive mindset, you will choose to go in the way that moves you forward, enabling you to make the changes you need to make. This is how you will grow and live a vibrant life.

Persistence and determination are the keys to following your dreams. My Swiss-German grandfather dreamed of building a cabin in South Lake Tahoe one day, but he knew it would be challenging. Yet, he saved his money to purchase the land and pursue his dream.

He built the place he envisioned. There was no lumberyard nearby, but that didn't stop him. He faced the challenges head-on, and every weekend, he drove to the site carrying lumber in his truck to build his cabin. He was persistent and never gave up, and eventually, he achieved his dream. Why? Because his mind was open to possibilities, and failure was not an option. He taught me the same principle, and I have lived my life with the same determination.

Ask yourself – are you determined enough to build your dream? To keep at it until it's completed? My dad was this person. Despite having his own physical struggles, my dad persevered through it all to achieve his goals.

My Dad's Struggle

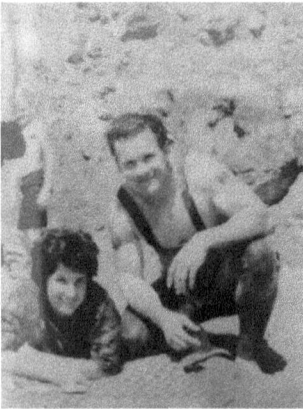

Gari M. Sommer,
circa the early 1960s

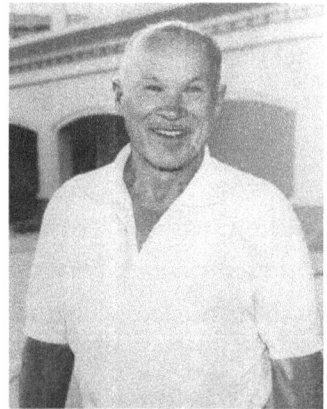

My Dad in his 70s.

To help you understand my perspective, I will start with my dad's story. Growing up in Cleveland, Ohio, he was surrounded by nature. One thing he loved was soil and tractors. He loved farming and seeing things grow, especially things he attended and cared for. Unfortunately, he was born with a bad leg. His left leg would often swell up with pain and stiffness, stifling his ability to enjoy his childhood. He often found himself bedridden for months. One day, he was reading a magazine article about Bernard McFadden, a mentor he looked up to and followed, born in the 1800s. Bernard McFadden was trying to create a movement of health and wellness in the American people by eating a healthy diet, weightlifting, and even entered in the American strong man movement.

My dad was particularly impressed by one article. It was about Bernard MacFadden strong and healthy, and jumping out of planes. Why did this impress my dad?

Not because he wanted to jump out of a plane, but because he couldn't understand how a man Bernard's age could be strong enough to do that. Bernard had the energy to do whatever he wanted to do. My dad took it to heart and realized he could change his life if he changed his mindset. His appendix burst when he was a child on the way to the hospital in a snowstorm. It was a horrible life-threatening experience, but he made it to the hospital on time. After getting out of the hospital, he knew he never wanted to see the inside of a hospital again. He was determined to strengthen his mind and body. He got up and never gave up.

He eventually even found and connected with his estranged biological father, whom he had never met. His dad had moved to California, and soon after they met, he realized his father had a very poor diet and was aging at an accelerated rate. One day, he found his father on the floor, dead from a heart attack. He was only 58 years old. While it was a huge shock for my dad, it made him realize once again that he needed to persevere and lead a healthier lifestyle.

He met one of the first gym owners in Sacramento and was encouraged to begin working out with weights. He eventually was encouraged to enter the Mr. Sacramento competition and came in 2nd place. He beat the odds. He was told years earlier that he would never walk normally and would spend much of his life in bed and in pain. Yet, here he was, overcoming his own struggles by eating healthily, exercising daily, and training to become strong.

"If we change the formula, no matter what it is, it will change everything. Even a one degree of change will result in greater life or faster death."
Scott Sommer, LAc

Legends of the Past
(Jack LaLanne, My Dad's Mentor)

No matter who you talk to, whether they are high-performers or not, they all start somewhere. Some people like me, my father, and my grandfather, were born sick, weak, and beat the odds. The fundamental difference between a successful person and an unsuccessful person is the successful person continues to push through doubt and discouragements as they work toward their goals with unwavering determination and persistence. Successful people seek mentors to guide them in their pursuits.

As I mentioned, my dad was born with a weak leg, which was his life's achilleas heel.

While his first mentor was Bernard MacFadden, he also discovered Dr. Bernard Jensen, Adelle Davis, Paul Bragg, and Jack LaLanne. Jack LaLanne and his wife, Elaine, were the first to have a fitness show on TV showing people how important it was to be fit, strong, and eat a healthy diet. Jack once admitted that, as a kid he was "a sugar Holic and a junk food junkie." He said, "It made me weak, mean, and sick; I had boils, pimples, and was nearsighted. Little girls used to beat me up. My mom prayed. The church prayed." Then, he met Paul Bragg, who changed his way of thinking. Through his own struggle, he embraced a new mindset and changed his life. His philosophy was simple – it is easy to die, and sometimes living is just a painful experience.

But you can do it. You can live a disciplined life. All you must do is eat right, exercise daily, and treat your health account like your bank account. Make daily deposits and invest in your future by being on the offense of potential physical problems – the more you put into it, the more you get out of it. Exercise and nutrition are the keys to living a long, vibrant, healthy life, which begins with the right mindset.

He focused on the benefits of eating the right food. Before Richard Simmons and Jane Fonda promoted health and fitness, the world already recognized Jack LaLanne for his public lectures on health, fitness, and nutrition, with dozens of books under his belt. These books and his TV show influenced people like my dad and me to follow in his footsteps and believe we could do anything we set our minds to.

The Power of Influence

Bernard McFadden, Dr Bernard Jensen, and Jack LaLanne greatly impacted their followers. Their enthusiastic and positive mindset affected people worldwide and persuaded them to become all they could be. You may be down and out right now, but if you embrace a positive, hopeful, and enthusiastic mindset, you will begin to bloom in ways you never imagined. You can choose which voices to listen to when your mind is open. You can choose to listen to those living the life you desire, or you can choose to listen to the negative voices in your midst. You will become like the 5 people you surround yourself with the most. They will define your emotional, spiritual, and physical perspective. It is up to you to choose a life-or-death mindset. "Bad company corrupts good morals," but bad company will also define your future. If you surround yourself with people who think 50 is old and arthritis, diabetes, and high blood pressure just come with age, then you can bet you will develop these conditions.

Yet, if you surround yourself with enthusiastic, motivated, self-disciplined people who think 50 is the new 30, you, too, will be enthusiastic, motivated, and self-disciplined. You must find a mentor and surround yourself with the right people to sustain a positive mindset. If you want to change your life for the better and become strong, fit, and healthy, you will be drawn to those who influence you in that direction.

The human mind is powerful, and having a positive mindset encourages us to take risks, to be bold, and to have the confidence we need to surpass any problem we face. We can climb any mountain and overcome any obstacle in our way if we believe we can.

Western Medicine vs. Eastern Medicine

Western medicine looks at your body with a limited mindset. It focuses on blood tests (which only show 7% of what is going on in the body), symptoms, and surgery. Using pharmaceutical drugs to treat most conditions. Resolving one issue while creating five more.

The concept of ancient medicine is a whole-body mindset. It's looking at the trees closely while seeing the entire forest at the same time. Interpreting how they influence each other. This is my approach when I meet a new patient. I look at their condition or diagnosis determined to find the root cause. Considering all contributing factors that led to this point. Western medicine has its purpose and its place, yet it fails to look for the root cause. Ancient medicine goes back 5000 years, and the results speak for themselves. If a patient comes to my practice not fully understanding what we do and has a level of hesitancy, I encourage them to read the reviews and do their research. The power lies in the testimony of others.

Testimonial

Scott Sommer, LAc
Sommer's Holistic Health Center

Sommers Holistic Health Center has been beyond amazing. Over years, visiting the Center to deal with post-cancer challenges, burnout, anxiety, and depression. Scott has worked with me and helped me to understand and overcome my health problems. I am renewed and reinvigorated for life.

My wife and I have recommended Scott Sommer to many people with wonderful health results. One of the greatest stories is our daughter's ability to conceive after years of trying without any success. Within a short time after visiting the Center and sticking to the prescribed process, we now have five grandchildren.

Scott has been a dedicated learner of the human body for many decades. His continuous dedication to growth is an inspiration and motivation to grow myself.

I highly recommend Scott Sommer's Natural Life Center. It is absolutely worth it, and you will see awesome results.
–Joe Antekeier

What Motivates People to Change?

This is one of the oldest questions asked, and there is no right or wrong answer. Some may say their motivation is money, power, material goods, or fame. These may be instrumental in the outcome, but they are external motivators. The best motivation comes from within, the place where our inner drive and feelings rule, which will ultimately determine our decisions in every area of life. Your success will be as great as your desire, and that applies to your health as well as your position in life. If you desire to change and grow, then you will seek out those people and things that inspire you and help you to change and grow.

Most people are motivated to change something when they feel pain or discomfort, whether it be financial, emotional, or physical, it pushes them to do something about it. For example, if you have a serious health issue, you may reach a critical point and realize you must make a serious change to your eating habits and lifestyle to fight against the diagnosis or condition. If you are poor, you experience hardship and know the only way out is to work hard and make the money necessary to dig yourself out of the hardship. You must make one critical decision before you can make the next. Remember, this is not permanent; it is just a speed bump in the road, a challenge you must embrace. A mountain you must climb.

You must envision yourself free of pain and leading the life you've always wanted. Believing in your heart that if you make the necessary changes and do what you need to do, your life can be restored to what it was before your condition or situation took over. Sometimes, the pain and discomfort will open your mind to the possibilities before you. Knowing things can absolutely be different if you work hard. Once you realize the possibility exists, you can pray about it and plan to change. Once you envision this you will have the motivation to change and become the best you can possibly be.

We only get one shot at life, and it's time to take control. Become the best you and leave behind a legacy you can be proud of.

Success Story

Before seeing Scott, I had high blood pressure, acne, fatigue, poor eyesight, and uncontrollable sweating. After seeing Scott, I realized that my blood pressure is normal, I have clear skin and great eyesight, I no longer sweat excessively, and I'm full of energy.

When I first came to Scott, I believed that my health issues were bad luck and genetics. I believed that the only option I had was to manage them with pharmaceutical medications and treatments. Scott opened my eyes to the fact that all health issues can heal with a proper lifestyle, nutrition plan, and connection to nature. Scott taught me the fundamentals of natural health that have helped me achieve a state of perfect health.
–Riley Check, Age 24

Books to Read to Improve Your Mindset

- Who Moved My Cheese by Spencer Johnson, MD
- The Five People You Meet in Heaven by Mitch Albom
- Atomic Habits by James Clear

- The Power of Focus by Jack Canfield, Mark Hansen, and Les Hewitts
- 7 Habits of Highly Effective People by Steven Covey

Chapter 2

Water

"In the beginning, God created the heavens and the earth.
Now the earth was formless and empty, darkness was over the surface
of the deep, and the spirit of God was hovering over the waters."
–Genesis 1:1

From the beginning, water was the foundation of life. There is a sequence to creation and an ancient pattern for us to follow: water comes before life can begin.

Water is the key to life, and hydration is one of the most important parts of health and wellness.

In the beginning, we were cocooned in water in our mothers' wombs. Every cell in our body was formed and encased in water. Before we are born, the water breaks, and we come forth to take our first breath. Yet, our reliance on water doesn't end when the sac breaks.

The human body is made up of 50% to 60% water.

- The brain is 85% water
- Blood is 83% water
- The heart is 79% water
- Bones are 22% water
- Muscles are 75% water

- The liver is 85% water
- Kidneys are 83% water[1]

This is astounding, isn't it? Dehydration affects our organs, bones, and brain. If we lack water and are dehydrated, we will suffer in multiple ways, both physically and mentally. Every day, we lose 8-12 cups of water from respiration, skin, urination, bowel movements, and other bodily functions alone.[2]

The Effects of Dehydration

Dehydration is serious. Many people think they get enough hydration by drinking tea, coffee, juice, or soda throughout the day, but it's not the same thing. You need water.

Have you ever wondered why you get headaches? Do you find yourself struggling to think clearly as the day goes on? Ask yourself how many times you urinate during the day and what color it is. When you're hydrated, you will urinate every couple of hours. If you only go twice a day, you are not getting enough water. You aren't getting enough water if your urine is dark and strong-smelling. Your argument might be, "If I drink enough water, I will spend all day in the bathroom, so not drinking water saves time." That's a valid argument, but remember, everything comes to a standstill when you don't drink water. If you live in a hot climate, drink alcohol, or

---

[1] "The Water in You: Water and the Human Body," The Water in You: Water and the Human Body | U.S. Geological Survey, accessed July 15, 2024, https://www.usgs.gov/special-topics/water-science-school/science/water-you-water-and-human-body#:~:text=According%20to%20Mitchell%20and%20others,bones%20are%20watery%3A%2031%25.

[2] Allie Wergin, "Water: Essential for Your Body," Mayo Clinic Health System, April 17, 2024, https://www.mayoclinichealthsystem.org/hometown-health/speaking-of-health/water-essential-to-your-body-video#:~:text=Every%20day%2C%20you%20lose%20eight,a%20minimum%20of%20nine%20cups.

consume caffeine, you will suffer even more from dehydration. If you persist in not drinking enough water, dehydration's short-and long-term effects can be painful. Take a look at the table below.

Short-Term Effects	Long-Term Effects
Persistent headaches	Increased urinary tract infections (UTI) and kidney stones (dry kidneys)
Fatigue	Hypertension (Thick blood)
Brain fog	Dementia (Dry Brain)
Constipation	Constipation (Dry Colon)
Weight gain	Decreased kidney function and potential kidney disease
Dry mouth and dull, moisture-less skin	Wrinkles, cracked skin, swollen tongue, tongue sores. Decrease in saliva, increase of bacteria and gum disease.

Scared yet? If the short-term effects of dehydration don't motivate you to drink more water, then the long-term complications should.

How Water Works in the Body

The earth needs water to survive, and so do we. Our blood runs through our veins and is dependent on water. Too little water and our blood slows down, becomes sluggish, and heightens our risk of blood clots. When we eat, stomach acid breaks down the food, but our body needs water to push the food through our digestive system. Otherwise, it sits in the colon and rots. When we urinate, toxins are released from our bodies. We must drink enough water to urinate every couple of hours. This ensures harmful toxins are being released from our bodies. Your liver and kidneys filter your blood and dispose of toxins. Water takes toxins out of your body. When you don't drink enough water, your liver and kidneys can't do their job, and toxins remain in your body. This soon leads to the build-up of toxins, constipation, and infections. Common problems with the digestive system, UTIs, kidney stones, and other kidney infections are often caused by a lack of water.

Principle: Ancient History

Ancient medicine was developed by humans making keen observations of nature, including plants/herbs, animals, seasons, and everything related to the earth. They observed how our bodies interact with the Earth because we were created from the Earth. For example, in ancient medicine, too much water in the body in one area is called dampness. This term would equate to water retention, swelling, hypertension, candida or yeast, etc.

What Kind of Water?

That might seem silly, but drinking enough water isn't enough – it must be the right kind of water.

Tap Water: No matter how clean you think your tap water is, you must avoid drinking it. It's full of chemicals, fluoride, and heavy metals, none of which are good for you. Aside from the metals and chemicals in tap water, other things can find their way into it as well. Researchers have found several other chemicals, including prescription medications such as antibiotics, antidepressants, contraceptives, and so on.[3] Steroids found in the water are known to cause infertility and other problems in fish. When people urinate, they release toxins from their bodies, but they also release remnants of the medication(s) they take. The water is sent to a sewage center, where it is cleaned and recycled. Remember, when you run a glass of water from the tap, you are potentially drinking someone else's heart, blood pressure, thyroid, or even hormonal medication.

If tap water is your only option, then invest in a water filtration system which has at least a five-stage filtration system. The water runs through a filter and cleans out the sediment, heavy metals, and contaminants.

Bottled Water: You might think bottled water is healthier, but it can be worse. When plastics break down over time, they can form smaller particles called microplastics, which are 5 mm or less in length – smaller than a sesame seed. Microplastics, in turn, can break down into even smaller pieces called nano-plastics, which are less than 1 mm in size.[4] Unable to be seen with the naked eye, these are small enough to enter the body's cells and tissues. Previous research has found evidence of plastic particles in human blood, lungs, gut, feces, and reproductive tissues like the placenta and testes. However, the potential health effects of these tiny plastic bits are still unproven and unknown.[5] These plastic particles leach into the water and mimic estrogen in the body, which can lead to competition between hormones, a hormonal imbalance, and weight gain.

---

[3] Roger Collier, "Swallowing the Pharmaceutical Waters," CMAJ : Canadian Medical Association journal = journal de l'Association medicale canadienne, February 7, 2012, https://www.ncbi.nlm.nih.gov/pmc/articles/PMC3273502/.

[4] "Plastic Particles in Bottled Water," National Institutes of Health, January 30, 2024, https://www.nih.gov/news-events/nih-research-matters/plastic-particles-bottled-water#:~:text=T.

[5] "Plastic Particles in Bottled Water," NIH.

Distilled Water Removes Minerals From Water: Adding liquid minerals is necessary to get these minerals back. We sell liquid minerals which is a fantastic way to supplement distilled water.

Natural Spring Water is the closest to its natural form, so it is the best water to drink if filtered. I recommend Reverse Osmosis (RO) filtration systems.[6] According to the Environmental Protection Agency (EPA), the RO process "forces water through a semi-permeable membrane under pressure, leaving contaminants behind."[7] The RO technique requires considerable water pressure to overcome natural osmotic pressure and effectively remove impurities and harmful particles.

Water pH

What does pH have to do with the water you drink?

Theoretically, our blood should have a pH of around 7.35 to 7.45[8], although some parts, like the colon and digestive system, need to be slightly more acidic. If the pH levels drop below 6.9 in the blood, it can lead to a coma. The pH level is maintained in the body using primarily three mechanisms: buffer systems, respiratory control, and renal control.[9]

---

[6] Aquasauna reverse osmosis filters can be found here: https://www.aquasana.com/.
[7] Overview of Drinking Water Treatment Technologies," EPA, accessed July 15, 2024, https://www.epa.gov/sdwa/overview-drinking-water-treatment-technologies.
[8] Noreen Iftikhar, "What's a Normal Blood ph and What Makes It Change?," Healthline, August 16, 2019, https://www.healthline.com/health/ph-of-blood#p-h-scale.
[9] Dr. Surat P, "Ph in the Human Body," News Medical, October 10, 2022, https://www.news-medical.net/health/pH-in-the-Human-Body.aspx#:~:text=pH%20indicates%20the%20level%20of,is%20critical%20for%20their%20function.

So, should you spend extra money on alkaline water to keep your pH at the right levels? No, avoiding acidic foods and eating an alkaline diet is better at managing your pH. An exception is some foods that are acidic but become alkaline upon digestion, such as lemons. I suggest adding organic trace minerals that we use in my practice to make the water slightly alkaline.

Distilled water

The problem with distilled water is that it removes the minerals your body needs. You must supplement your diet with minerals to ensure you are getting enough in your system, but you can also purchase mineral drops for this purpose. You can order this product from our clinic or add a pinch of salt to your water, such as Redmond Real Salt®. Many of the Pink Himalayan salts come from China and are riddled with chemicals, so do your research.

Healing the Body with Water

Dr. Bateman, an MD, was in a Middle-Eastern concentration camp. He had little at his disposal to help people who were sick or suffering to get better, so he started to study how water affected the human body and certain conditions. He treated a range of conditions – asthma, fatigue, constipation, and so on – and he discovered that water could help improve, if not reverse, each condition. And that's what he did – he cured thousands of people with nothing more than water.[10] So, what does that tell you? It tells us that water has power beyond anything we've ever known. It tells us if we drink enough water every day, we can overcome certain conditions we already have

---

[10] F. Batmanghelidj, Water: For Health, for Healing, for Life: You're Not Sick, You're Thirsty! (New York: Grand Central Life & Style, 2012).

while also preventing others from developing in the first place – there's nothing more powerful than that.

We are all guilty of thinking the worst when we don't feel well. Most of us resort to pharmaceuticals or complicated solutions when natural, simple solutions exist. Did you know you can go for weeks without food but can only survive a few days without water? Most of us drink something every day, but not drinking enough water is very detrimental to our health. Your bones dry out, and you damage your liver and kidneys. That's why so many elderly people get UTIs in their later years; Most do not drink enough water. Their urinary tract is clogged with sludge and riddled with yeast, leading to chronic kidney infections.

Let me give you another example of how important water is to your body. Try washing your car with coffee, juice, or soda and see what happens. Of course, you can't wash it; you would end up with a stained, sticky mess while also ruining the paint. If you had used water in the first place, your car would have sparkled and shined. The same thing happens to your body. Fill up on caffeine, juice, and soda, and your body and skin will become a hot, gloppy mess full of substances that suck the water right out of your system. Fill up on clean, life-giving water, and your body will thank you. Washing your car is like washing your body – do it right the first time, and the results will speak for themselves.

Hungry or Thirsty?

Not drinking enough water can also cause weight gain. When you feel hungry, or your blood sugar is too low, you are most likely thirsty. You might not feel thirsty, but a hunger sensation can be one of the first indicators that you're dehydrated. Instead of reaching for a snack, drink a glass of water and wait. If you still feel hungry after 20 minutes, then it is true hunger, but most of the time, one glass of water will do the trick.

Many people don't realize that when they awaken in the morning, they are already dehydrated. Your body loses water while you sleep through sweating and even through breathing. The first thing you should do when you get up in the morning is to drink a 32 oz jar or glass of warm water with lemon. Drink it straight down and get that water flowing back through your body. Many people believe that cold water is better, but it isn't. Water must be as near to your body temperature as possible to do any good.

Drink another large glass of water 20 to 30 minutes before every meal. Not only will you feel better at the end of the day, but you'll also eat less, and that is great news for those who want to lose weight! Doing this ensures your body has sufficient water to digest the food, move the toxins out of your body, and feed your cells with the water they so desperately need. Imagine that without water, your cells dry out and can't function properly

Simple Ways to Tell If You Need More Water

- Monitoring the color of your urine – it should be straw-colored. If it is darker and has a strong smell, you aren't drinking enough.
- Pinching your skin – good, hydrated skin will spring back instantly, while dehydrated skin is dry, papery, and sluggish.
- Dizzy and lightheaded? There's a good chance you need more water.
- Is your mouth dry? Drink more.

- Head aching? Drink a glass of water.
- No energy? Constipated? You know the answer.

Everything begins with water and ends with water. Think of a plant. It doesn't matter how much soil, fertilizer, and sunlight you give it; it cannot survive without water. Now think of your body – you can give it food and sunlight, but it cannot survive without water. The less water you drink, the less your cells get, and the harder it is for them to do their jobs. Every cell in your body affects your organs, so with less water, your organs suffer. If your liver, kidneys, heart, and digestive system don't work as they should, the risk of disease is so much higher.

The next time you feel hungry between meals, drink water. Don't reach for a sugary soda to cool down or a cup of coffee for a shot of energy. Soda, sugar, and coffee pull the water out of your body (they are the enemies of good health). Only water can save you.

Think about what staying hydrated will do for you. The more water you drink, the less pain you will have because it lubricates your joints, tissues, bones, and brain. H2O also helps regulate your bowels, while giving you energy and oxygen. It is life-changing to embrace water as a daily priority. Water is the spice of life, the only way to ensure your health and happiness. Lastly, picture a field in your mind, in the sun without water for months. Picture it. Brown, dry, and dusty. Then, picture it as the rain begins to fall on the field. Watch it as it turns green and bounces back to life. That is what water does to your body.

Testimonial

Scott Sommer doesn't simply treat symptoms. He sets out like a seasoned investigator to target the source of the problem. He sees the "whole person" and helps him/her heal with nutritional advice, help with staying hydrated, whole food supplements, essential oils, natural products, cutting edge services and apparatuses along with sound coaching for life practices that allow healing to happen. I highly recommend his unique practice and services.

–Therese Tiab

Here Are Some Great Ways to Stay Hydrated

1. Buy yourself a 40 oz Stanley or a Hydro Flask on Amazon. Drink 3 of these a day. Morning, noon, and night. As my wife tells my patients, "Just suck it down, concentrate on it, and do it."

2. Embrace the challenge of drinking a minimum of at least half your weight in ounces of water each day, but as stated above, 120 oz works the best.

3. Start your day with a lemon sliced and squeezed into 32 oz. of warm water or hot water with green tea or energy tea. Another drink I recommend to all my patients is the SHOVEL drink I created 20 years ago (salt, honey, olive oil, apple cider vinegar, and lemon). Each drink will help hydrate and detox the body daily. Stay away from sugar laced drinks which spike blood sugar and do not hydrate the body.

4. The best water filtration system is a 5-stage filtration system, or a reverse osmosis system in which you must add minerals.

Final Thoughts

"Water is the mirror that can show us what we cannot see. It is the blueprint for our reality, which can change with a single, positive thought. All it takes is faith if you're open to it."
–Dr. Masaru Emoto[11]

Water may seem like such a simple thing, but it is the most vital aspect of our health and survival. Most of us greatly underestimate the fact that every cell, bone, organ, and tissue depends on water. Without water, we age at an accelerated rate, we get wrinkles, our hair becomes dry and thin, and our body decays (unnaturally) simply because it is dying for water. A body without water is like a car without oil. A few days without water leads to brain fog, tiredness, and a lack of energy. When you skimp on water, you will suffer from the above.

Scan the QR Code with your Smartphone
to view message about What Water Does to Our Body.

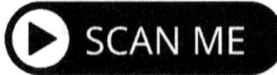

Or follow this link: https://qrco.de/whatwaterdoestoyourbody

---

[11] For further reading about Dr. Emoto https://www.alivewater.ca/.

Chapter 3

Your Immune System is Your Fortress

"I want to praise you because I am fearfully and wonderfully made."
—Psalm 139:4

What is your immune system? It is composed of the bone marrow, thymus, spleen, lymph nodes, and various components of the mucosa-associated lymphoid tissue (MALT). The immune system organs are immature at birth and develop over the first 6 weeks of postnatal life and beyond.[12]

The immune system can also be likened to a castle with high walls around it and a moat of water around it to protect you, the walls being likened to your skin. The openings are the sinus, mouth, and skin. In theory, the immune system should defend you by preventing unwanted and dangerous guests from crossing the castle's moat into the body. However, sometimes it doesn't work the way it should. The aim of this chapter is to describe how the immune system works, how it fails, and how you can strengthen it, so it functions properly.

Ask Yourself These Questions:

- How many times a year do you get sick? Do you recover quickly?
- Do you have seasonal allergies or year-round allergies?

---

[12] George A. Parker, Tracey L. Papenfuss, in Atlas of Histology of the Juvenile Rat, 2016.

- Do you have food allergies or an auto-immune condition?
- Do you have digestion issues such as chronic diarrhea, bloating, constipation, or IBS?
- Do you suffer from skin conditions such as eczema, psoriasis, rosacea, cracked hands or feet?
- Are your nails cracked, split, spotted, or have fungus?
- Is your tongue coated in the morning? Is it cracked? Or pealed and shiny?
- Do you have chronic sinus congestion or sinus infections?
- Do you snore?
- Cold Sores, Canker Sores, or Pink Eye?

You must ask yourself these questions and understand why these are all signs and symptoms of a weak immune system. The most common drugs used in response to these immune system conditions are antibiotics, antifungal, antiviral, or antiparasitic. We must look at the root cause of why our immune systems are weak and out of balance. Ancient medicine looks at the connections and root causes of the imbalances in the immune system and finds safe and natural solutions, such as food, plants, nutrition, lifestyle, and detox, instead of drugs and surgery. These should only be used rarely and as a last resort. You must consider *why* you are on medications and why you began experiencing these symptoms. Why do so many suffer from these common conditions?

You may run to Western medicine, submit to random tests, receive a diagnosis, and do exactly what the doctor says. Yet, we know the medications only lessen or alleviate the symptoms, while each has side effects. Most doctors are uneducated in nutrition because medical schools do not teach it. They don't look for the root cause of your symptoms or tell you how to change them because they simply do not know. They have been trained to treat symptoms. They use pharmaceuticals, surgery, or physical therapy to treat problems. Yet, the answer lies in strengthening our immune system.

A Weakened Immune System

The immune system is like airport security. No one should get on a plane that doesn't deserve to be there, especially if they have weapons of mass destruction. This is like a bomb getting past airport security and making its way onto the plane. When security is down these unwanted terrorists sneak on the plane to carry out their plan. Once they have control of the plane, they can do as much damage as they want. This is what happens to our immune system when it's weak. It allows unwanted bacteria, viruses, or parasites into the body, where they can wreak havoc on the whole operation.

The Fires

How do we get sick? To explain this, I'll use a fire metaphor. We all know where there's smoke (symptoms), there's fire (sickness or disease). The big question is, what causes it, and where did the smoke come from? Well, there's often more than one factor, and it can be difficult to figure out how the fire started without looking at the warning signs that something isn't right – headaches, brain fog, insomnia, and many others indicate that something is off balance. God created our bodies to send these warning signals to us so we can look for the root of the problem and resolve it naturally.

While a medical diagnosis may point to a specific problem, sickness reveals your immune system has been compromised. The complex network of systems that keep your body running are simply unable to function when stressed by an improper diet, lifestyle, stress, or unclean environments (mold, dust, or EMFs).

You must search for the "why" before you can fix the "what." This is always the first step in determining what the plan should be. This is the objective of Holistic Medicine.

Types of Immune Challenges

- **Bacteria** are microscopic, single-celled organisms that exist in the millions in every environment, both inside and outside other organisms. Some bacteria are harmful, but most serve a useful purpose. They support many forms of life, both plant and animal and are used in industrial and medicinal processes. Bacteria are thought to have been the first organisms to appear on Earth. The oldest known fossils are of bacteria-like organisms. Bacteria can use most organic and some inorganic compounds as food, and some can survive extreme conditions. A growing interest in the function of the gut microbiome is shedding new light on the roles bacteria play in human health.[13]

  Most people believe that antibiotics will knock out a bacterial infection. Yet, it isn't always the case. Many bacterial infections are complex, sometimes consisting of several infections at once. Viral infections are untouchable and do not respond to antibiotics.[14] Bacterial infections were discovered in the 1600s with the invention of the microscope. These infections require special attention, but with a strong immune system, most people recover quickly. Our immune system determines our outcome.

---

13 "Bacteria," Encyclopædia Britannica, July 15, 2024, https://www.britannica.com/science/bacteria.

14 "Healthy Habits: Antibiotic Do's and Don'ts," Centers for Disease Control and Prevention, accessed July 15, 2024, https://www.cdc.gov/antibiotic-use/about/index.html.

- **Viruses** are microscopic particles in animals, plants, and other living organisms. They can sometimes cause diseases, such as the flu and COVID-19. Viruses are biological entities that can only thrive and multiply in a host (a living organism such as a human, an animal, or a plant). Some viruses cause disease. The same virus can affect different organisms in different ways. This explains why a virus that causes illness in a cat may not affect a human. Viruses vary in form and complexity. They consist of genetic material, DNA or RNA, with a protein coat around it. Some have an additional coat called the envelope. This may be spiky and helps them latch onto and enter host cells. They can only replicate in a host.

- **Parasites** live in other host organisms and depend on them for survival. Parasites that can affect humans include ticks, lice, and hookworms. Symptoms of a parasite infection in humans can vary widely. A parasite cannot live, grow, and multiply without a host. For this reason, a parasite rarely kills its host, but it can spread diseases, some of which may be fatal.

After 25 years of clinical practice, I've seen many patients that are riddled with parasites. They often experience serious digestive issues, which Western medicine often calls **irritable bowel syndrome** (IBS). Parasites rob your body of nutrients and leave behind waste. One source of parasites is contaminated food such as sushi, farmed-raised fish, pork, contaminated water, soil, and even people. Common fish carry parasites (such as roundworms and tapeworms) that are a danger to humans if ingested.[15] So, make sure

---

[15] "Illness Causing Fish Parasites (Worms)" (British Columbia: Canada, January 2013).

to thoroughly cook your fish before consuming it to kill bacteria and parasites.

Possible Symptoms of a Parasitic Infection Include:

- Neurological problems like seizures or severe headaches
- Skin bumps or rashes
- Weight loss, weight gain, increased appetite, or both
- Abdominal pain
- Diarrhea and vomiting after travel or the avoidable foods.
- Sleeping problems

How to Prevent Parasitic Infections

- Avoid eating raw sushi, pork, and farm-raised fish.
- Avoid sitting on a public toilet.
- Make sure your pets/animals are dewormed. Do not let them lick you.
- Avoid drinking contaminated water, in other countries, especially in Mexico, South America, and Africa.
- Avoid swimming in polluted ponds and lakes.

Overactive Immune
Allergies or Auto-Immune

Food allergies are becoming incredibly common worldwide. According to the Asthma and Allergy Foundation of America (AAFA), more than 100 million people experience various types of allergies each year, and we know that allergies are the 6th leading cause of chronic illness in the U.S.[16]

---

[16] "Allergy Facts," Asthma & Allergy Foundation of America, April 19, 2024, https://aafa.org/allergies/allergy-facts/.

You may not know you have an allergy to food, but you may have constipation regularly. You may feel bloated, have gas, or suddenly find you lack energy. It may come right after a meal or the next day, but you can't tie it to anything in particular. The one dead giveaway is feeling extremely tired right after a meal – a reaction to a type of food you ate. In some cases, a food allergy presents itself almost immediately, with a rash, itching, swelling, or, in some extreme cases, anaphylactic shock, which is incredibly life-threatening. Even mild food allergies can cause serious conditions, such as celiac disease or bleeding in your gut. One of the biggest contributors to food allergy-related diseases is gluten, found in wheat-based products and many other foods. Gluten sensitivity is one of the most common allergies, causing significant discomfort in the gut and disrupting your digestive system, leading to constant discomfort, diarrhea, constipation, indigestion, and many other symptoms.

Celiac Disease is caused by an abnormal immune response in genetically susceptible individuals triggered by ingesting gluten proteins from wheat, rye, and barley.

Airborne Allergies

Airborne allergies include tree pollen, grasses, pet hair, dust, mites, fungal spores, and other airborne allergens. These include industrial and food allergens, which often circulate during food preparation. Seasonal allergic rhinitis is an allergic reaction to pollen from trees, grasses, and weeds. This occurs primarily in the spring and fall when pollen from trees, grasses, and weeds is in the air.[17]

---

[17] "Allergy Facts," AAFA.

Airborne Allergy facts

- While exact numbers are challenging to obtain, experts estimate that 30-40% of the world's population has allergies.[18]
- Airborne allergens are the major cause of allergic rhinitis and asthma. Daily exposure comes from indoor sources, chiefly at home but occasionally at schools or offices.[19]
- In 2021, approximately 81 million people in the U.S. were diagnosed with seasonal allergic rhinitis (hay fever). This equals around 26% (67 million) of adults and 19% (14 million) of children.[20]

Allergy symptoms manifest in several ways: itchy red eyes, sneezing, coughing, wheezing, struggling to breathe, fatigue, and just not feeling well. Most people experience these when in an environment they may be allergic to. In my practice, we can clear these allergies through what we call an *Allergy Clearing*.

Mycotoxins and Mold Allergies

Mold is a type of fungus. In general, normal amounts of mold in the environment do not pose a substantial health risk to healthy people with regular immune system function. There is no single "black mold" type – many molds are black. When people use the term, they may be referring to Stachybotrys chartarum (S. chartarum), also

---

[18] Dave Davies, "Why Our Allergies Are Getting Worse -and What to Do about It," NPR, May 30, 2023, https://www.npr.org/sections/health-shots/2023/05/30/1178433166/theresa-macphail-allergic-allergies#:~:text=Estimates%20are%20that%2030%20to,U.S.%20and%20around%20the%20world.

[19] Peden D;Reed CE;, "Environmental and Occupational Allergies," The Journal of allergy and clinical immunology, accessed July 15, 2024, https://pubmed.ncbi.nlm.nih.gov/20176257/.

[20] AAFA.

known as Stachybotrys atra. However, some people may be more sensitive to mold spores than others and may develop respiratory symptoms after inhaling even a small number of spores. Those with an allergy or sensitivity to the spores may experience symptoms such as congestion, red eyes, respiratory problems, and skin rashes. In large quantities, mold spores can cause ill health in almost anyone.[21] Therefore, people should remove any mold growth in the home and take steps to prevent it from growing back.

Many people have mycotoxins and yeast in their bodies caused by exposure to mold, sugar, candida, and lack of water. They are produced by molds (fungi) and can accumulate in crops, posing health hazards to humans and animals. According to the USDA, Mycotoxins are estimated to affect 25% of the world's crops.

Environmental Allergies

Do you find yourself reacting to the clothes you wear or touch? Do you ever develop a painful or itchy rash? Get migraines? Do you find that your eyes are achy, and you feel tired? That can be a reaction to environmental allergens commonly used on new clothing. Although harmful chemicals are everywhere, new clothing is one of the most toxic items you will likely encounter. They are full of dyes, formaldehyde, flame-retardants, and more.

Many Americans have allergic reactions to environmental allergens at work. In fact, exposure to unusual substances at work can cause occupational asthma, accounting for approximately 5% of asthma in adults. Some 12.6% of Americans report hypersensitivities

---

[21] A Bitnun and R M Nosal, "Stachybotrys Chartarum (Atra) Contamination of the Indoor Environment: Health Implications," Paediatrics & child health, March 1999, https://www.ncbi.nlm.nih.gov/pmc/articles/PMC2828207/.

to common chemicals.[22] Is it unlikely that some people are more sensitive to certain exposures than others?

People who are extra sensitive to EMFs (electrical, magnetic fields) often suffer from other kinds of allergies, too, such as food, environmental, and airborne. These effects are often hard to pinpoint because they surround us daily, but there are ways to be on the offense. One is buying an Energy Mizer for your home. This device plugs into your electrical outlet at home and absorbs much of the EMFs coming into the home or out of the plugs in your home. I will list the resources for these items at the end of the chapter.

Strengthening Your Immune System

Let's go back to the 1900s, when the great flu pandemic swept the world, and ask yourself the same question being asked today about the COVID-19 pandemic – why are some people getting sick and dying while others appear untouched? The answer lies in our immune system. Knowing and understanding the signals your body is sending is vital to resolving many of these issues. Educating yourself is the first step to getting better. When you know more, you do more.

I've seen countless patients in my own medical practice get off pharmaceutical drugs simply by changing their lifestyle and diet. My patient, Dusty, was struggling with a weak immune system that led to long Covid. Here is his story.

---

[22] Stanley M Caress and Anne C Steinemann, "Prevalence of Multiple Chemical Sensitivities: A Population-Based Study in the Southeastern United States," American journal of public health, May 2004, https://www.ncbi.nlm.nih.gov/pmc/articles/PMC1448331/.

Testimonial

I was very weak with long Covid and had been seeking answers/ treatment with medical specialists (cardiologist, pulmonologist, gastroenterologist) for a full year. I'd had five miserable ER visits when I set up my first appointment with Sommer's Holistic Center. I was too weak to drive, too dizzy to stand up, and could not complete a sentence without stopping to breathe. The brain fog was horrifying and had been increasing for a full year since the COVID-19 infection. I could not tolerate noise, sunshine, or social contact. My gut was cramping and in distress and had been for years. As a 72-year-old lifelong competitive endurance cyclist/runner, I was non-functional and desperate for help.

Within days of my first visit with Scott, I started feeling more clear-headed. My brain fog receded, and my lifelong gut issues have gone away. What a relief – I could run my own errands! And go for short walks! Now, at 6 months out, I'm running twice a week, and going for 50-mile bike rides again! I'm calmer than I have ever been in my life. I think more clearly, and I'm both serenely happy and fully energized. My creative energy is back, and I've been making commissions again.

Along with that, my CT scan shows that my lungs have recovered (the scarring is no longer there), and my workout stats are showing an increase in fitness. Scott asks questions and LISTENS to my answers. His positive energy and intuition are a huge benefit. His office is staffed with kind and professional therapists who offer encouragement and understanding, and the numerous therapies offered are helping me recover. I am extremely grateful that I found Sommer's Holistic Center.
–Dusty, Age 72

Tips to Strengthen Your Immune System

- Examine your life (past and present) to understand what may have affected you in the past and what is affecting you now so you can make the necessary changes to improve your immune system and feel your best.
- Ditch the elevator, car, bus, or train and start taking the stairs, walking, or riding a bicycle.
- Eat clean – embrace nutritious whole foods as medicine to your body.
- Stop turning to prescriptions and over-the-counter medications and find out about healthy alternatives.
- Take lysine If you have cold sores or herpes (HSV). Studies show that it helps with outbreaks and flare-ups.[23] Lysine is found naturally in some foods, such as beef, eggs, and yogurt. It can also be found as a supplement or cream. Ask your physician about dosage. Don't use lysine if you are pregnant.
- Avoid ultra-processed sugars such as corn syrup or white sugar, brown sugar… etc. There's always a substitute that is better for you and tastes just as good. We recommend alternatives like stevia, honey, maple syrup, maple sugar, date or coconut sugar, and monk fruit.
- Avoid genetically modified (GMO) foods (learn more about GMO in chapter 4).
- Invest is whole food supplements – we use Standard Process that has been available since 1929.

In summary, we are sick because we have weak immune systems. A lack of exercise, insufficient water, poor diet, too much sugar, and

---

[23] Anthony, Kiara. "Lysine for Cold Sores: Treatment, Risks, and More." Healthline, March 13, 2023. https://www.healthline.com/health/lysine-for-cold-sore.

poor dental hygiene may lead to health problems. It is a vicious cycle, right? A poor diet and stagnant circulation are often the root of common conditions and terminal or chronic diseases.

In our next chapter, we will discuss how your diet makes you sick and how to fix it.

Scan the QR Code with your Smartphone to view message about the IMMUNE SYSTEM.

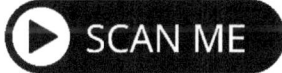

Or follow this link: https://qrco.de/ImmuneSystem

Chapter 4

Food and Digestion

The food you eat has a significant effect on your health. Western medicine will tell you it has nothing to do with your symptoms, but it does. When you ask them *why* you have certain symptoms, they can't give you an answer. Yet, a poor diet is often the primary cause of disease. Ever wonder what the difference is between people who are overweight and those who aren't? Many people carrying extra weight also suffer from brain fog and difficulty sleeping. When you're overweight, you have a higher risk of diabetes, cancer, and heart disease.

- Are you struggling to think clearly?
- Is it hard for you to keep your skin clear?
- Struggle to stay active?
- Have pain but can't pinpoint the cause?

It all comes down to the food disease pipeline, starting with the farm.

The Soil

My dad always told me, *"The secret is within the soil."* Over the last century, modern farming practices have contributed to a lack of nutrients in the soil. The food grown is only as good as the soil it is grown in. For example, studies show that magnesium deficiency can be attributed to common dietary practices, medications, and farming techniques, along with estimates that the mineral content of vegetables has declined by as much as 80–90% in the last 100 years.[24] The soil has been stripped of its natural nutrients and minerals. In addition to this, the crops are often heavily sprayed with pesticides, fertilizers, insecticides, and weed killers – you name it, they use it. We weren't designed to consume harmful chemicals.

The only solution to this problem is to buy organic foods as much as possible, go to farmer's markets, or start growing your own food. Home-grown and organically grown vegetables often have more flavor than mass-produced vegetables in stores. If you garden at home, you can plant what you want to eat in nutrient-rich soil. Even if you only have a small space, you can grow many delicious vegetables in containers and planters on your patio or back porch. To avoid using harmful pesticides, try companion planting. This helps to keep beneficial insects that are so important to our food while keeping the bad bugs away.[25] Pull weeds by hand without weed killers, and your health will repay you in spades.

Bread is a staple food that once gave life but is now causing many health conditions. Did you know that the healthiest part of the wheat plant is the wheat germ? In the old days, when wheat was ground to make flour, the wheat germ was ground with it, making bread an incredibly healthy food. These days, our bread is made from GMO wheat with few nutrients, and the wheat germ is removed to stop the flour from turning rancid. The process of commercial

[24] Workinger, Jayme L., Robert. P. Doyle, and Jonathan Bortz. "Challenges in the Diagnosis of Magnesium Status." Nutrients 10, no. 9 (September 1, 2018): 1202. https://doi.org/10.3390/nu10091202.

[25] Benedict Vaheems, "Companion Planting Chart and Guide for Vegetable Gardens," Almanac.com, June 5, 2024, https://www.almanac.com/companion-planting-guide-vegetables.

breadmaking makes bread worthless with no nutritional value. Not only do they remove the wheat germ and wheat germ oil with the very beneficial vitamin E, but they also bleach it, removing all nutritional value. Then, they add synthetic vitamins to replace all the nutrients they just removed. The problem is that the body may not properly absorb synthetic vitamins and nutrients. The corporations making bread do not care about your health. They simply add the nutrients to the labels, so it makes people feel better about buying it. There are no nutritional benefits when eating this manufactured bread. It turns into sugar and robs the bones of calcium. Learn how to make your own bread by searching YouTube for tutorials, or you can also invest in a bread maker. Whatever you can do to accomplish this would be a game-changer in your home. Learning these skills and taking hold of your health is vital. If you can't possibly make bread, buy it carefully and look at the labels. If you're going to eat bread, eat sprouted bread or Ezekiel bread. Ezekiel bread is primarily made from legumes and organic wheat.

Making Healthy Choices: Too Much Highly Processed Food

Think about your average trip to the store. Is your cart filled with highly processed foods and junk? The difference between processed and unprocessed food is unprocessed food comes from a garden, orchard, or farm straight to your home or to the store. Processed food is any altered fruit, vegetable, or food item that has been cleaned, dehydrated, cooked, juiced, or frozen like tofu or canned vegetables. There are good organic frozen berries and vegetables, but you need to look at the labels. Ultra-processed foods have added oils (soybean oil, vegetable oils, canola oil), corn syrup, salt, sugars, fats, preservatives, MSG, and artificial colors. Many manufactured foods have additives that affect your health in a negative way.

Highly processed foods lack fiber, have too much sodium and sugar, and are riddled with chemicals and synthetic vitamins. Fiber is what keeps your digestive system functioning as it should and regulates your blood sugar. Many processed foods cause constipation, and inflammation in the body. A lack of fiber leads to many complications with your digestive system, but also causes diabetes, cancer, and heart disease.[26] When you consume these foods, you may develop stubborn belly fat which is hard to lose. This creates insulin resistance and digestive problems. Which we will talk about later in this chapter.

A Vicious Cycle

The Agricultural Industry, the Food Industry, and the Pharmaceutical Industry are all trying to sell you something. They make you sick, addicted, and dependent. The sicker you are, the more money they'll make. How? For example, you go to the doctor with digestive issues, diabetes, heart disease or cancer. They put you on medications to alleviate the symptoms, but do not resolve the problem. I call it the perfect set-up. Then, the side effects begin, causing a multitude of other problems. It is a vicious cycle destroying lives. Cancer is the biggest money maker of them all, and when you consume these foods long enough, the chemicals and additives cause cancer.

The 2024 Dirty Dozen

Each year, The Environmental Working Group (EWG) publishes the "Clean 15" and "Dirty Dozen" lists to help consumers make

---

[26] "Health Benefits of Dietary Fibers Vary," National Institutes of Health, June 21, 2022, https://www.nih.gov/news-events/nih-research-matters/health-benefits-dietary-fibers-vary.

informed choices when they shop for produce.[27] The list indicates which crops tend to be treated with the highest volume and variety of pesticides but doesn't go so far as to say which ones are the riskiest from a human health perspective.

Here is the most recent list:

- Strawberries
- Spinach
- Kale, collard, and mustard greens
- Grapes
- Peaches
- Pears
- Nectarines
- Apples
- Bell & Hot Peppers
- Cherries
- Blueberries
- Green Beans

More than 50 pesticides were detected on samples from each item on the Dirty Dozen, except cherries. And all of the produce on the Dirty Dozen had at least one sample with at least 13 pesticides – and some had as many as 23.

---

[27] Emma Loewe, "Update: The Dirty Dozen & Clean 15 Lists for 2024 Just Dropped," mindbodygreen, April 3, 2024, https://www.mindbodygreen.com/articles/ewg-dirty-dozen-and-clean-15-lists.

The 2024 Clean 15

As is the case every year, you'll notice that most of 2024's "cleanest" produce has a tough outer peel, husk, or shell that is removed prior to eating. Makes sense!

- Avocados
- Sweet corn
- Pineapple
- Onions
- Papaya
- Sweet peas (frozen)
- Asparagus
- Honeydew melon
- Kiwi
- Cabbage
- Watermelon
- Mushrooms
- Mangoes
- Sweet potatoes
- Carrots

Almost 65% of Clean Fifteen fruit and vegetable samples had no detectable pesticide residue.

America – The Sumo Wrestler

Let me give you an example of a sumo wrestler. Their primary goal is to be as heavy as possible and to beat their opponents on the mat. The heavier and stronger they are, the better chance they have of winning. It comes down to their diet. Most choose to eat extensive amounts of unhealthy carbohydrates.

If you want to be as big as a sumo wrestler then eat a high-carb diet consisting of unhealthy carbohydrates. This would include white rice, pasta, pizza, bagels, bread, and many kinds of heavy, carbohydrate-rich foods. They do one thing – push your blood sugar level through the roof and spike your insulin. Many patients come to me desperately wanting to lose weight or stop gaining weight, unsure of what to eat and what not to eat. We've been conditioned to eat these things, and as a result, many are suffering from obesity. Think about the grain-fed farm animals. They are much fatter than their healthier, grass-fed counterparts. The same happens to you – if you eat grains all day, every day, you too will gain weight and be obese.

Now, let's add some trans fats to those carbs, like French fries. They are just carbohydrates fried in trans fats. In fact, any deep-fried food is loaded with trans fats, and when added to the high amounts of unhealthy carbohydrates, you will have the perfect recipe for a sumo wrestler.

The body requires food for fuel. It is our source of energy. It enables us to do everything we need to do with the right amount of food and water. The primary fuel source is glucose, or blood sugar, which we get from carbohydrates, which turn into sugar in your blood. However, your body can only burn so much, so when you overeat, the excess sugar is immediately stored as fat, usually settling around your major organs and in your belly.

So many people eat large, fatty, carb-laden meals throughout the day and do little to no exercise. In this country alone, 75% of the American population is classified as overweight. Obesity in children has become an epidemic because our households are filled with chips, soda, ice cream, alcohol, fried foods, white bread, and rarely fruit and vegetables.[28] All of these things contribute to obesity. When we bring these foods into our homes, our children eat them and become addicted to salt and sugar too.

Then, as adults are trapped in their own bodies and unable to shed weight, we must stop the cycle and turn the tide by embracing the colors of the rainbow diet, which I will address in the next paragraph. In addition to these vibrant fruits and vegetables, you must include protein. If you can, I would encourage you to eat organic beef bison, lamb or wild-caught fish, and legumes. There are tips on what to eat later in this chapter.

How do you stop this? How do you stop being a sumo wrestler and become a toned athlete?

By cutting unhealthy carbohydrates and ditching processed foods for good. Athletes eat a good amount of carbohydrates but burn them off through exercise. For a sedentary lifestyle, the same amount of carbohydrates is unnecessary and can impact your health.

Chicken

You might think chicken is the healthier choice but unless you raise your own free-range chicken. The chicken you buy in stores is full of chemicals, antibiotics and hormone. These accelerate the growth of the chicken. Even the organic choices are questionable simply because the standards for organic are so minimal when it comes to chickens. They are injected with extensive antibiotics regularly because there are thousands of sick chickens crammed together in pens.

---

[28] National Center for Biotechnology Information accessed July 22, 2024, https://www.ncbi.nlm.nih.gov/.

Then antibodies are put in their food to counteract the effects of antibiotics and to stop them from spreading disease between one another. If you want to improve your health and lose weight, avoid eating meat that is full of hormones, chemicals, and antibiotics. Estrogen is one of the main components in chicken, which is responsible for breast cancer, and other cancers.

What is White Trash?

White trash is white flour, sugar, dairy, and refined salt consisting of bread, donuts, bagels, and cakes. We discussed processed breads in the beginning of this chapter.

Dairy: Added hormones and antibiotics are dangerous for your health. Yet, they are added to all dairy products simply to keep the milk flowing. All milk-based products have hormones. Cream (coffee creamer, salad dressings, cheese, and yogurts). Cows are saturated with antibiotics, just like chickens, to keep the infection from spreading between one another. Many are sick because they are injected with so many chemicals. The best dairy would be organic or raw milk, sheep or goat or European cheeses.

Sugar: It's a time-bomb waiting to wreak havoc on your body. The more sugar you consume, the worse you feel. Excess sugar creates inflammation in the body, and inflammation is one of the main contributors of disease. It causes your blood sugar to spike and crash, spike and crash. Do you know what that means? Your body wants to eat more sugar to raise your blood sugar again to get that burst of energy back. It's a vicious cycle – the more sugar you eat, the more sugar you want, and the sicker you get. Studies have shown that it is more or as addictive as cocaine.

Sugar is big business here in the United States and around the world. It has a long and brutal history.

Did you know that Christopher Columbus brought sugar cane to America on his second voyage to the New World in 1493?[29] Then, colonists, traders, and merchants planted it all over the West Indies and throughout South America. Indigenous and African individuals were enslaved and forced to work in brutal conditions on sugar plantations while white traders and industrialists got rich. From there, it was eventually processed into refined sugar, and the downward spiral began. From this brutal history, we moved into the modern era when technology made producing and refining sugar easier, and manufacturers and producers began adding sugar to food.

Now, sugar is included in almost all processed foods. To hide it they have renamed it on labels, and now there are up to 75 different names for sugar. Making it very difficult for the average shopper to recognize. Yet, you must know and recognize these names to avoid sugar. It is the most addictive ingredient in food, and the primary cause of obesity and disease. Sugar is acidic and leads to heart disease by creating plaque in the arteries, fatty liver disease, diabetes, obesity, acne, eczema, and many other conditions. Sugar feeds cancer and helps it to grow. That is why they do PET scans. They send radioactive glucose through your veins to identify where the cancer cells are, because cancer cells love sugar and absorb 60x more of it than non-cancerous cells. When you eat sugar, it damages your immune system for 5 hours. A study was done in 1970 and again in 2011 by Loma

---

[29] "The Sugar That Saturates the American Diet Has a Barbaric History as the 'white Gold' That Fueled Slavery." The New York Times Magazine, August 14, 2019. https://www.nytimes.com/interactive/2019/08/14/magazine/sugar-slave-trade-slavery.html.

Linda University,[30] found that as little as 75 grams of refined sugar or high fructose corn syrup, which is equivalent to a cupcake, 24 oz of soda, sweetened yogurt, or a sports drink is like leaving the front door of your house open for 5 hours, and allowing anyone to come in. According to Ancient medicine, it creates dampness (candida) in the body, and weakens the digestive power of the spleen (pancreas).

Whole foods and a Mediterranean diet stabilize our blood sugar, but a standard white trash American diet spikes our blood sugar. Our blood sugar is the lifeline to our immune system. Inflammation, heart disease, non-alcoholic fatty liver cancer, energy, sleep, and life itself are all fueled by our blood sugar. In essence, it is our vitality. If you suffer from one of the above, give up refined sugar and white trash.

Where sugar was once a delicacy or condiment, only available to the rich, we now consume, on average, 150 lbs. of sugar per person per year. The next time you go to the grocery store, head straight to the sugar aisle and put 120 lbs. of it in your cart. Just look at it. If it doesn't make you feel sick, just thinking about that much sugar consumed by your body in one year, then you must be incredibly addicted to it. Many resort to artificial sweeteners like sucralose, aspartame, or saccharin, and even stevia as a replacement for sugar. Yet, each of these spikes your blood sugar and causes glucose intolerance. Glucose intolerance prevents the body from going into ketosis, which is why people who use these artificial sweeteners can't lose weight. Artificial sweeteners also cause an imbalance in the gut biome.

---

[30] "Lick the Sugar Habit Book by Nancy Appleton," ThriftBooks, November 27, 2003, https://www.thriftbooks.com/w/lick-the-sugar-habit_nancy-appleton/253596/#editi on=1543011&idiq=1289680.

Flour: While whole grains contain three components – bran, germ, and endosperm – refined flour is made from grain that has been processed to remove the bran and germ, as mentioned above, leaving behind the starchy endosperm, which is pulverized into flour. The high starch content of refined grain and lack of fiber due to removing the bran and germ produces a rapid increase in blood sugar when consumed. The hyperglycemic and hyperinsulinemia effects of refined flour can cause severe blood sugar swings, which over time can significantly increase the risk of chronic diseases such as type 2 diabetes and cardiovascular disease.[31]

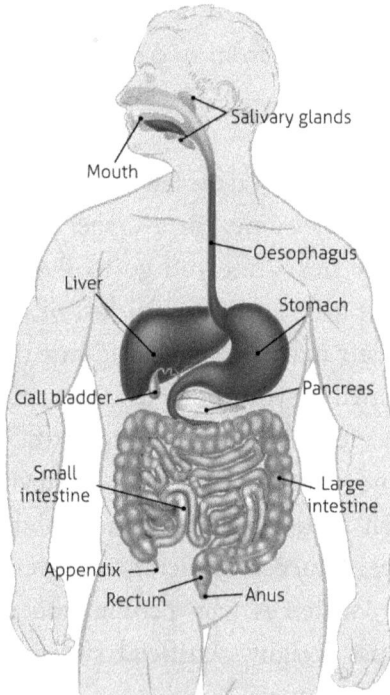

The digestive system (image by Clker-Free-Vector-Images from Pixabay)

---

[31] Heather Hall et al., "Glucotypes Reveal New Patterns of Glucose Dysregulation," PLOS Biology, accessed July 22, 2024, https://journals.plos.org/plosbiology/article?id=10.1371%2Fjournal.pbio.2005143.

How often do you think about your digestive system? It is usually when it gives you trouble.

It is one of the most misunderstood processes in the body, and it causes the most problems. So, I want to break digestion down into three parts.

The digestive system is like a factory conveyor belt. You start at one end with a product, and by the time it gets to the other end, it's an entirely new thing. So, let's start at the very beginning.

What You Consume

Food and drink provide nutrients, vitamins, and minerals needed to give us energy and to help our bodies restore and repair. Much of our lives revolve around food, and we should absolutely enjoy our food as it is one of the joys of life. Most of us spend much of our time eating with friends and family. We have taste buds to know what we like and don't like. They give us the desire to eat, leading us to chew and swallow the food, sending it on a journey through the digestive system. The ability to smell food is also important, as it can kickstart the whole digestive process. Smelling and chewing food helps produce saliva from salivary glands. It is an important part of the digestive process. We also have another gland in the mouth – the parotid gland.

This gland is incredibly helpful in two ways – digestion and detox. Believe it or not, when you chew your food, you also begin a detoxification process. Chewing efficiently causes digestive enzymes to be released, which help break down the food from something we can't use into something we can.

Nutrition from whole foods and wholefood supplements is the body's currency, and everything else aside from water is considered counterfeit currency. You can't build a healthy, vibrant body on counterfeit currency because your nutritional economy will crash into disease. You can't fool your body with synthetic spin-off vitamins and minerals. These are counterfeit and made in a laboratory. Food grown on depleted soil or sprayed with toxic chemicals is ruining your health.

Where the Food Goes

When you chew your food and swallow it, it goes down into your stomach, and this is where the magic starts to happen. The stomach's muscular walls mix food with hydrochloric acid and enzymes. Imagine the food in your stomach as being like clothes in a washing machine. After about an hour of digestion in the stomach, all the nutrients, amino acids, fatty acids, fiber, and carbohydrates are broken down into something called liquid chyme. Like detergent and softener, the liver and gallbladder then produce bile, which is alkaline with a ph of 7 to 8.6, to neutralize stomach acid, which is released into the small intestine and helps break down the fats, and promotes detox of unwanted toxins. Meanwhile the pancreas releases insulin into the bloodstream and enzymes into the small intestine to break down carbohydrates and balance blood sugar.

Principle

Our digestion is like a snowman. Each part leads to the next. Every part must complete its job, or you will end up with an incomplete digestion cycle causing gas, bloating, constipation, anemia, acid reflux, diarrhea and ultimately fatigue and exhaustion from a malnourished body and leaky gut.

The Intestinal Process

The small intestine is a bit of a misnomer because it really is quite long. When the digested food enters this long hose coiled in your body it absorbs what it can use. The nutrients are absorbed back into your blood which moves to your liver where it is then converted into something else.

Everything passes through your liver and continues its journey down 30 to 35 feet of the intestine, where it enters the large intestine, which is about 12 feet long. From there, what your body doesn't need is excreted out. From start to finish, like a spin cycle on a washing machine, the entire process is like a separation cycle, as it keeps the nutrients and disposes of the toxins from the body. The food is separated into what you need and what you don't need and then ends in the elimination process. The surplus fiber and other nutrients are then passed out of the body.

When the digestive system is doing its job, we don't even notice the difficult work it is doing to sustain our energy and keep our bodies functioning. All is well. But what happens if you start having problems? How can you figure out how to fix what went wrong?

What Went Wrong?

All sorts of things can go wrong with the digestive system, and it doesn't have to be complex. It can be as simple as not having enough teeth in your mouth to chew your food properly or simply swallowing food whole because you can't be bothered to chew it. Believe it or not, that can significantly affect the digestive process. First, you don't get all the nutrients you need from the food, and second, unchewed food is harder for your body to digest, which can lead to constipation, one of the biggest indicators that your digestive system is malfunctioning.

The next place things can go wrong is in your stomach. Some people suffer from belching, acid reflux, heartburn, stomach acid, or bad breath within 20 minutes of eating something. This indicates an upper GI (gastrointestinal) problem rather than a lower one. If you are bloated, have gas, or are distended, this indicates a lower GI problem.[32] Much of this is because you simultaneously eat the wrong combination of foods, (i.e., slow and fast-digesting foods). Fats take much longer to digest than some fruits and carbohydrates, which move through our digestive system quickly, like sodas and other high-sugar drinks.

Food combining is very important.

Here are the Four Most Common Rules of Food Combining

1. Always eat fruit, especially melon, on an empty stomach. Or at least twenty minutes before eating anything else.

2. Eat starches alone or with cooked non-starchy vegetables.

3. Eat meat, dairy, fish, eggs, and other high-protein foods alone or with cooked non-starchy vegetables.

4. Eat nuts, seeds, and dried fruit with raw vegetables.

---

[32] "Heartburn and Acid Reflux." NHS. Accessed July 19, 2024. https://www.nhs.uk/conditions/heartburn-and-acid-reflux/#:~:text=Causes%20of%20heartburn%20and%20acid%20reflux&text=certain%20food%20and%20drink%20%E2%80%93%20such,indigestion%20and%20heartburn%20in%20pregnancy.

Many people have gastrointestinal disorders that are present with symptoms like bloating, constipation, gas, and diarrhea. About 20% of adults will deal with irritable bowel syndrome (IBS) during their lifetimes. This is a painful condition that causes both diarrhea and constipation.[33] I've seen patients over the years who look and feel like they are pregnant, yet they are just full of gas due to their diet and eating habits. If you consume dairy, you may have gas and bloating. This can only be eliminated with the right foods, enzymes, and prebiotics.

Digestion problems don't just affect your gut, though. They also affect your hair, skin, nails, and energy levels and interfere with your ability to get a good night's sleep. When your diet lacks good protein, amino acids, and cleansing foods that clear the liver out, your digestive system can't function properly.

You Are What You Eat

You must pay attention to your digestive system. What you eat and how you eat it are important factors because if your body cannot digest food properly, you will have painful digestion issues, many of which are uncomfortable. It's simple – if you cannot digest your food properly, you will always have problems with your digestive system.

---

[33] Dr. Liji Thomas, MD. "Irritable Bowel Syndrome (IBS) Food Triggers." News-Medical.net, September 2, 2022. https://www.news-medical.net/health/Irritable-Bowel-Syndrome-(IBS)-Food-Triggers.aspx#:~:text=Bloating%20due%20to%20bacterial%20fermentation,in%20altering%20normal%20gut%20metabolism.

How Does It Work?

If you do not chew your food properly, it confuses the digestive system and stops it from producing sufficient enzymes to break the food down fully. This leads to:

- Diarrhea
- Heartburn
- Acid reflux
- Bloating
- Headaches
- Nausea
- Stomach cramps
- Irritability
- Indigestion
- Skin, hair, and nail problems
- Malnutrition

Here Are the Solutions

Chew your food: On average, you should chew each bite about 30 times – softer foods require less chewing, and harder foods require longer. Chewing your food this long will break it down and change its texture. It also makes digestion easier.

Don't drink fluids with your meal: Wait 30 minutes before or after eating, but never with your food. Also, do not drink iced or cold drinks, which can slow the digestive system.

Drinking warm water or tea before you eat: This prepares the stomach for its work, helps absorb the nutrients in your food, and helps prevent bloating, gas, and that heavy feeling after eating.

Choose herbal teas, like cinnamon, fennel, ginger, and lemon, as they help heat the body, invigorate it, and promote healthy digestion. In our clinic we carry a variety of fantastic teas.

Fruits should be eaten separately: Part of this is because they digest faster than other foods. It is best to consume them before you eat your main meals of the day. They can move through your system without getting stuck behind slower-digesting foods and fermenting in your stomach. Plus, research shows that eating fruit before a meal can help your body limit the absorption of simple sugars, in turn reducing the glycemic index of what you eat.

Examine your tongue in the morning: In Chinese Medicine we look at the tongue to reveal or confirm the condition of our digestion, blood and organ toxicity.

TCM TONGUE DIAGNOSIS
ORGAN SYSTEM MAP

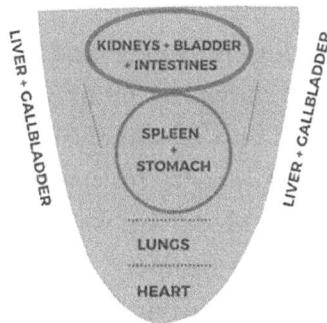

The tongue is a reverse map of the torso of the body. The tip of the tongue represents the heart, lungs, and emotions. The center of the tongue represents the digestive system. The sides of the tongue represent the liver and gallbladder. The base of the tongue represents the kidneys, bladder, and intestines. We use the appearance of the tongue in each section to give us information about the health of each organ system.

For example, a thick yellow coating at the base of the tongue may indicate chronic constipation or a bladder infection. A red tip of the tongue in the heart area may indicate anxiety or insomnia. A vertical crack in the center of the tongue may indicate digestive weakness.

TCM Tongue Diagnosis Examples:

- **Tongue body color:** This shows the circulation of Qi and blood. For example, a very pale tongue may be a lack of Qi like in chronic fatigue or lack of blood like in anemia. A purple tongue may indicate chronic pain or poor blood circulation.
- **Tongue shape and size:** The tongue should fit in the mouth without swelling and pressing into the teeth. We often see teeth mark indentations in the sides of the tongue, which tells us that the digestive system is weak.
- **Tongue coating thickness and distribution:** A thick white tongue coating can mean retention of fluids in the body or a build-up of pathogens such as yeast/candida. Alternatively, no tongue coating or a peeled coating can show a lack of fluids or what we call "yin deficiency" which is often seen in menopause.
- **Color of tongue coating**: A yellow coating can show a buildup of heat in the body or in a specific organ. Too much heat in the liver area can sometimes mean liver disease or alcoholism.
- **Tongue moisture**: The tongue should not be overly wet or too dry.

- **Tongue papules or cracks**: The tongue should be free of purple spots, red dots, or little cracks.

Eat the Rainbow

Fill your plate with color which will be enough fiber (25 to 30 grams a day). One big salad a day. Colorful foods, like squash, carrots, beetroots, peppers, oranges, blueberries, and so on, can help protect your body. Colorful foods are full of vitamins and minerals, while white trash has no nutritional value and causes bloating, weight gain, and disease. Eat local organic and seasonal foods, and you will experience benefits you never imagined. It's about what you eat. It's about the right amount of protein, a minimum of 25 to 30 grams at each meal, or even more if you are an athlete or want to lose weight, good fats for the brain and joints), and nutrients. The six essential nutrients are vitamins, minerals, protein, fats, water, and carbohydrates. People need to consume these nutrients from dietary sources for proper body function.

One of the best diets in the world is the Mediterranean diet (often called the Blue Zone diet). Make the switch from simple carbohydrates to complex carbohydrates like sweet potatoes, fruit, vegetables, and whole grains such as quinoa, buckwheat, or Ezekiel bread. Even if you don't have a garden, you can still grow your own vegetables and fruits in planters on your porch or patio. You can also get great, pesticide-free produce and support a local farmer by joining a CSA (Community Supported Agriculture) or visiting farmers' markets. Choose organic foods, grass-fed meats, free-range poultry and eggs, and wild-caught fish.

The food you eat is directly responsible for how well you feel. If you eat junk, you might feel good for a moment, but an hour or two later you will start to feel sick, heavy, and bloated. Do this on a regular basis and you will begin experiencing health issues, poor skin, lack of mental clarity, and in many cases even develop a serious disease related to your digestive system. According to a study on the role of nutrition in chronic disease, poor diet can lead to "cardiovascular disease, hypertension, stroke, type 2 diabetes, metabolic syndrome, some cancers, and perhaps some neurological diseases.[34]

> *"Illnesses do not come upon us out of the blue.*
> *They are developed from small daily sins against nature.*
> *When enough sins have accumulated, illness will suddenly appear."*
> –Hippocrates

And what about drinks? A sugar-laden can of soda, or a tall glass of sparkling clean water? Caffeine and milk-laden coffee or herbal tea? You don't have to drink plain water. Here are some ideas to make water more fun to drink:

- Add sliced fruits or vegetables and use them to flavor it,
- Add a few drops of apple cider vinegar.
- Add lemon to kick start your stomach acid and digestive juices, to aid with digestion.

Remember, you do have a choice. It all starts with your plate. Fill it with color. Colorful foods, like squash, carrots, beetroots, peppers, oranges, blueberries, and so on, can help you protect your body. Colorful foods are full of vitamins and minerals, while white trash has no nutritional value and causes bloating, weight gain, and disease.

---

[34] Gropper, Sareen S. "The Role of Nutrition in Chronic Disease." Nutrients vol. 15,3 664. 28 Jan. 2023, doi:10.3390/nu15030664

Live to eat or eat to live. You're the only one who can eat the right food. Be strong and stand alone in the presence of your family and friends to eat the life-giving foods and to live a vibrant life.

You will live longer if your diet is full of live food, clean food, and nutrient-dense food.

Tip:

Start renewing your mind with the following website: http://www.whfoods.org/index.php-
The 100 Healthiest Foods.
He has fantastic recipes and ways to get you started on your journey to health!

Reversing Disease with Food

Testimonial:

My 14-year-old son was diagnosed with IBD/Crohn's. Doctors from UCD told us that we have no other option than Remicade infusion. Went through infusion for about 6 or 7 months, but when we realized how harmful it was for his body, we started looking for a holistic doctor near us. After visiting Scott's office for about 3 months, my son feels so much better. He gained weight, ate with no restrictions, had no pain or diarrhea, good appetite, and felt like a normal teenager. We are so happy that Remicade is left behind forever. Thank you so much for helping us in our desperate situation.
–Tanya Lobkov

Helpful Tips for a Healthy Digestive System

- Drinking water or tea 30 minutes before or after a meal makes the digestive process more efficient.
- Never drink coffee right after a meal. It speeds up the digestive process, making it inefficient, and causes bloating and gas.
- Don't eat processed sweet foods or fruit right after a meal. Sugary foods digest much quicker and can cause bloating and gas.
- Do not partake in heavy exercise right after a meal. The digestive process needs energy, and if you use that energy to exercise, digestion slows and becomes inefficient.
- Include fermented foods in your diet, like pickles, kimchi, kombucha and sauerkraut. These are packed with natural digestive enzymes and plenty of beneficial bacteria that help the body absorb the essential nutrients in your food. If you eat fermented food daily, you can reduce the risk or symptoms of IBS, allergies, gluten intolerance, and asthma.
- Never boil your vegetables. When you eat them lightly steamed or raw, they retain fiber and enzymes, both of which are lost when the foods are boiled. Enzymes and fiber are required for successful digestion.
- Take a walk after a meal. This helps the food move through your stomach much quicker, thus helping the digestive system do its job.
- Take probiotics. When you don't sleep properly, or your eating habits are poor, your digestive system doesn't work properly. When you take a probiotic, you get a dose of healthy gut bacteria, which can help balance your gut biome. Call our office to get the best of the best or buy

good quality product with more than 30 billion from your local health food store.

- In the resources section of this book, you'll find a list of our favorite nutritious foods, recipes, and tips on eating. This is the list we give to our patients when they ask us, "What do I eat?"

- What you eat is also an important factor in digestion. Unhealthy fast foods, sugar-laden foods, processed foods, and heavy break or pastry-based foods take much longer to digest and sit in your system for longer. That leads to fermentation and causes all sorts of issues with your digestive system. When undigested food sits in your stomach, it stops other foods from being digested efficiently. Thus, you get a backlog inside you, resulting in great pain, discomfort, and feeling unwell. Stick to a healthy diet low in carbohydrates and high in healthy proteins and vegetables.

- Remember, digestion begins in the mouth. If you get off to a bad start here, it has a domino effect throughout the rest of your system. It impacts your health and the longer it continues, the worse your health problems become. The longer you have digestive problems, the greater the chance of serious disease later in life. If you insist on poisoning your body with a poor diet, then you can't expect it to repay you by staying healthy. You must give your body what it needs to survive and thrive. You can change your life by changing how you eat.

Only you can determine what type of life you want to lead. Only you can decide how healthy you want to be. If you want to be healthy, fit, and disease-free, watch what you eat and how you eat it. In our next chapter, we discuss healthy weight loss.

"There is no fountain of youth. What you put into your body is what you get out of it. You would not feed your dog a coffee and a donut for breakfast, followed by a cigarette, you will kill the damn dog."
–Jack LaLanne

"When a patient is struggling back up the mountain of health, I use the cycling phrase keep peddling. Once you stop peddling, everything stops, and you crash."
Scott Sommer, LAc

Scan the QR Code with your Smartphone
to view message about FOOD AND DIGESTION.

OR follow this link: https://qrco.de/food_digestion

Chapter 5

Weight Loss

Most of us are old friends with weight gain and weight loss. Some of us can maintain our ideal weight; others struggle to put weight on, while many people struggle to get rid of it. That final one is the biggest problem. Obesity prevalence among older Americans has increased at an alarming rate. According to the Population Reference Bureau, between 1988 and 2018, the share of obesity in U.S. adults ages 65 and older nearly doubled, increasing from 22% to 40%.[35]

Everywhere you look, you are bombarded with information about the latest celebrity diet or ads about other weight loss programs that, in all honesty, don't really work. Why? Because most of them are fads and are so restrictive that you just can't stick to them. Restrictive diets get boring, and what do most people do when they get bored? They eat. These diets are not sustainable. To a certain extent, portion control works. Most overweight people know that they are overeating or choosing unhealthy foods. They know that they binge eat, eat too much sugar, or eat too many highly processed foods. But there's more to weight than that.

The Weight Loss Wheel

Weight loss is complex, and being overweight is sign of a deeper problem. It comes down to a broken mechanism, something I like to call the Weight Loss Wheel.

---

[35] Mather, Mark, and Paola Scommegna. "Fact Sheet: Aging in the United States." Population Reference Bureau. Accessed July 19, 2024. https://www.prb.org/resources/fact-sheet-aging-in-the-united-states/.

The problem starts when a person wants to lose weight for various reasons. Maybe that's you. Remember when you felt like you were at the perfect weight and felt great about yourself?

When I've asked this question to many patients over the years I've discovered it is usually linked to something the patient used to do that was successful in maintaining a healthy weight. Yet, then something changed, and the patient stopped doing the successful action, so they no longer could maintain a healthy metabolism or a healthy weight.

This is a great lesson for all of us. When you stop doing what was working, then it just stops working. Sounds logical, right? Good health habits like exercising first thing in the morning or eating fruits and vegetables daily can be difficult to maintain after big life events.

Many men I've talked to say they used to go to the gym until they became a dad or work became more demanding. They stopped working out and stopped building muscle. For some women, they found it difficult to keep the weight off after they had children or hit menopause. Other tragic life events like a divorce, the loss of a loved one, or a big diagnosis can change your body and successful lifestyle habits. Think of it as being a row of dominos. When one falls, the rest follow. Everything starts with your emotions and stress, and then your digestive system. Stress is a big factor that causes excessive belly fat. The demands of working more, sleeping less, and eating on the run add to weight gain.

Many people don't like to admit they have succumbed to the culture and the way we eat. I will share some stats with you on the American diet – the biggest culprit in your weight gain, and in your inability to lose it.

Let's Look at the Five Spokes of Weight-Loss:

1. Food, Digestion and Insulin Resistance

Your weight is about what you eat, when you eat, the portion size, and how you digest your food. The main culprits in weight gain are bad carbohydrates, which lead to inflammation, insulin resistance, and body fat.

Four Food Options:

- Organic Whole Foods which are single ingredient foods.
- Foods processed with 3 to 5 ingredients.
- Highly processed foods with 15-35 masked chemicals and ingredients.
- Fast Food: high salt, high sugar, fructose, corn syrup, trans fats, and unknown dangerous ingredients like MSG, disguised by many names.

If you're an American, then option 3 would probably best define your diet, although if you're committed to your health, you probably avoid fast food. Option one will bring you a vibrant life, while those following will rob you of a vibrant life. It shows up in your joints, your belly, your muscles, and your bones.

The research bears this out. America's Health Rankings® Health Disparities Report reveals the urgent need to address maternal mortality, mental health, and food insecurity.[36] Many people find it hard to believe the U.S. performs poorly on most health measures

---

[36] "2021 Disparities Report: AHR," America's Health Rankings, accessed July 22, 2024, https://www.americashealthrankings.org/learn/reports/2021-disparities-report.

compared to other high-income countries. But the truth is, study after study supports the same two conclusions:

1. The U.S. spends more on health care but has worse health outcomes than comparable countries around the globe. This holds true across age and income groups.
2. Within the U.S., there are unacceptable disparities in health by race and ethnic group, county by county, and state by state.

High Spending and Poor Health Compared to Other Countries

Whether you measure health spending per capita or as a percentage of gross domestic product, the U.S. spends more than two times the average of comparable countries. A 2014 Commonwealth Fund report ranked the U.S. dead last against comparable countries for the fifth time in ten years.[37] That ranking was based on measures such as quality of care, access to care, equity, and healthy lives.

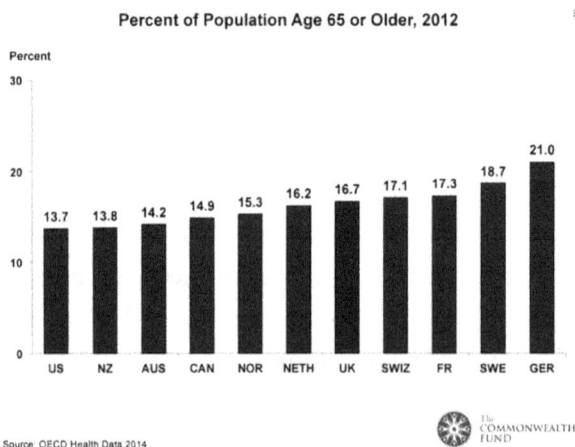

Percent of Population Age 65 or Older, 2012

Percent

Country	Percent
US	13.7
NZ	13.8
AUS	14.2
CAN	14.9
NOR	15.3
NETH	16.2
UK	16.7
SWIZ	17.1
FR	17.3
SWE	18.7
GER	21.0

Source: OECD Health Data 2014

The COMMONWEALTH FUND

---

[37] 2021 Disparities Report, America's Health Rankings

The Institute of Medicine looked deeply into U.S. health performance versus 16 of the most fairly comparable, high-income countries. Their study found that people in the United States have:

- **Shorter lives:** Over the past 25 years, U.S. life expectancy has grown, but at a lower rate than in other countries.
- **Bad birth outcomes:** We have the highest rates of infant mortality, low birth weight, women dying due to complications of pregnancy and childbirth, and children less likely to live to age 5.
- **More injuries and homicides**: Deaths from motor vehicle crashes, non-transportation injuries, and violence happen at much higher rates.
- **Heart disease**: The U.S. death rate from ischemic heart disease is the second highest. Adults over age 50 are more likely to develop and die from cardiovascular disease.
- **Obesity and diabetes:** For decades, the U.S. has had the highest obesity rate across all age groups, and American adults have high rates of diabetes.
- **Chronic lung disease:** Lung disease is more common in Americans and associated with a higher risk for death.
- **Disabilities:** Older U.S. adults report a higher prevalence of arthritis and physical limits to their daily activities.
- **Adolescent pregnancy and sexually transmitted disease**: Our youth have the highest rate of pregnancy and are more likely to acquire sexually transmitted diseases.
- **HIV and AIDS:** We have the second-highest prevalence of HIV infection and the highest incidence of AIDS.
- **Drug-related deaths:** We lose more years of life to alcohol and other drugs even when deaths from drunk drivers are excluded. In fact, the president's 2014 National

Drug Control Strategy noted overdose deaths surpassed homicides and car crash deaths.

While this sounds dire, the good news is that the public health community is already implementing programs to address these challenges.[38]

Fresh fruit, vegetables, and fiber-rich foods reduce appetite and detoxify the body. Eating more of these means eating less fatty, processed, and sugary foods filled with carbohydrates. The opposite of the keto plant-based diet is the American sumo diet – filled with fast food and grease – which is sadly the way many Americans eat. I believe that this trend started when fast-food restaurants started gaining speed. Also, portion sizes have increased over time and are out of control. Go to many fast-food restaurants, American cafes and eateries these days, and you'll notice huge meal sizes offered.

The average restaurant meal today is more than four times larger than in the 1950s

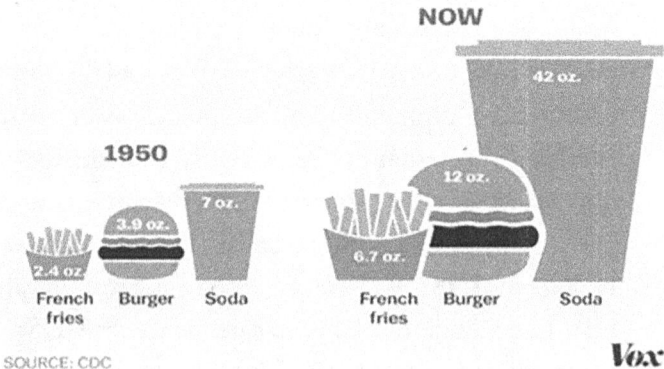

NOW

42 oz.

1950

12 oz.

7 oz.

3.9 oz.

6.7 oz.

2.4 oz

| French fries | Burger | Soda | | French fries | Burger | Soda |

SOURCE: CDC

Vox

---

[38] "Health Rankings." American Public Health Association – For science. For action. For health. Accessed July 19, 2024. https://www.apha.org/topics-and-issues/health-rankings.

In some cases, one meal would be enough to feed a whole family, yet one person sits and eats it by themselves. When you eat these foods, you run the risk of acid reflux. If your diet consists of high amounts of fast food, white flour, sugar, and dairy products, you can also expect problems with your digestive system. These foods are acidic and are considered unhealthy. When we were kids, eating pizza and drinking sugary soda was fine; we still woke up thin the next day. The older you get, the harder it

The Squirrel Effect

You might be amazed at how efficiently our bodies store fat. Just like a squirrel stores nuts for the winter, our body does the same. This happens when we eat too much food, eat too many carbohydrates, or if we eat at the wrong time of day – especially eating late-night meals. Our body stores the extra calories as fat since we're not using them. This is truly no different than a squirrel storing up food for the winter.

Your body was created for a purpose. That purpose to make a difference and contribute your gifts and talents to the rest of the world.

A squirrel stores its nuts to survive the winter or for a future event. You might start thinking about eating food to nurture, repair, and restore your body for the future instead of using it as a self-serving event, disqualifying yourself from a future event. Obesity and being unhealthy limit you from doing many things others can do effortlessly. Like picking up grandchildren, running in an emergency, sitting on an airplane, and playing physical games with your children. Being unhealthy robs you and your loved ones of many opportunities to create memories. So, over-eating and eating for pleasure can actually damage your daily life.

When you fill up your car with gas, it's like filling your body up with food. You either fill your body up with the right type of fuel or the wrong type of fuel. You can also try to fill the tank up too much so that it spills out on the ground.

Now, if this were your car at the gas station, you would avoid overfilling the tank because it would be a waste of money and make a mess. Well, this is exactly what happens to our bodies when we eat too much, especially when we eat the wrong foods. Such foods include simple carbohydrates, processed food, and white trash. You are spilling fuel on the ground and creating a mess that will be very hard to clean up.

When your weight loss wheel is broken, stressed, or bent, the weight simply will not come off. It's called **Metabolic Syndrome.** Metabolic syndrome refers to the presence of a cluster of risk factors for cardiovascular disease. Metabolic syndrome greatly raises the risk of developing diabetes, heart disease, stroke, or all three.

According to the National Heart, Lung, and Blood Institute (NHLBI),[39] the cluster of metabolic factors involved includes:

- **Abdominal obesity:** This means having a waist circumference of more than 35 inches for women and more than 40 inches for men. An increased waist circumference is the form of obesity most strongly tied to metabolic syndrome.
- **High blood pressure**: Is 130/80 mm Hg (millimeters of mercury) or higher. Normal blood pressure is defined as less than 120 mm Hg for systolic pressure (the top number)

---

[39] "What Is Metabolic Syndrome?" National Heart Lung and Blood Institute. Accessed July 19, 2024. https://www.nhlbi.nih.gov/health/metabolic-syndrome.

and less than 80 mm Hg for diastolic pressure (the bottom number). High blood pressure is strongly tied to obesity and is often found in people with insulin resistance.

- **Impaired fasting blood glucose**: This means a level equal to or greater than 100 mg/dL (milligrams per deciliter)
- **High triglyceride levels:** Of more than 150 mg/dL. Triglycerides are a type of fat in the blood.
- **Low HDL (good) cholesterol:** Is considered low when it is less than 40 mg/dL for men and less than 50 mg/dL for women.

Metabolic Syndrome makes you feel heavy, bloated, and slow. Acid reflux, bloating, diarrhea, constipation, and every other symptom of poor digestion will follow. You will feel tired, washed out, and generally unwell. When this happens, and there is no other reason for it, it is a clear indicator that your digestive system is in turmoil.

Fixing this requires help. Digestion starts by chewing your food slowly and long enough to help it digest, and you should not drink water or any other drink with your meal. Instead, sip a little water about half an hour before you eat and then wait an hour after eating before you drink anything else.

2. Your Liver, Gallbladder, and Detoxification

The second spoke on this wheel is your liver. Liver problems are indicated by bloating, constipation, and light-colored stools. The latter indicates that your liver and gallbladder (true partners in crime) are not producing enough bile or aren't flowing through them properly. The liver and the gallbladder are paired organs in Traditional Chinese Medicine. The liver produces bile, which flows down to the gallbladder so the gallbladder can digest fats and detoxify the body.

Clinically I have found the gallbladder is one of the most problematic organs when people are trying to lose weight. When the liver and the gallbladder are not working properly it is very hard to digest fat, and to lose your own body fat. When a person loses their gallbladder from surgery, it becomes very difficult to digest food or to lose weight. Irregular bowel movements, diarrhea, and constipation are all symptoms of an unhealthy liver and gallbladder.

The liver is like a factory where the bile is produced, but it does more than that; the liver has more than 500 functions, which means many of your symptoms may indicate an issue with the liver. For example, high cholesterol indicates inflammation somewhere in your body and this is linked to the liver. Airborne and food allergies are indicators that your liver is not functioning correctly. Food allergies are indicated by an intolerance to certain foods. You suddenly can't eat much, but what you do eat causes a reaction in your digestive system. This usually occurs when your diet consists primarily of fatty, greasy foods containing unhealthy seed oils. These can cause pains in your stomach or between your shoulder blades, indicating issues with your liver or gallbladder.

Eating fatty foods and feeling bad afterward indicates that your liver is struggling to detox your body. The same is true when your skin is suddenly full of blemishes and acne or when you notice eczema or psoriasis.

Signs that your body needs a serious detox are bloating, a general heavy feeling after eating, and when even drinking water makes you feel full. The human body removes toxins from the body in five ways:

How the Body Removes Toxins	Detox Suggestion
Skin (through sweating)	Infrared sauna or dry sauna
Feet	Epsom salt foot bath, Professional Grade Ionic Detox Foot Baths[40]
Bowel Movements (bile flows from the liver and gallbladder)	Ensure you're eating a healthy diet full of organic vegetables and fiber
Urination (kidneys filter toxins from the blood and expel them)	Stay hydrated
Breathing (exhaling expels toxins)	Daily activity and exercise

When your detox pathways are closed, your body becomes sluggish and weight loss becomes impossible. Keeping those pathways clear is easy – drink more water, eat more vegetables, eliminate white and brown sugar, and processed dairy products (cow) (replace with sheep or goat).

Your body should detox every day in some way. Many people find that intermittent fasting helps (only eating in a window of time

---

[40] "Vibrational Products – Learn, Comparisons, Testimonials, Resources." Hymbas. Accessed July 19, 2024. https://www.hymbas.com/vibrational-machines-resources.php.

like 12 pm to 6 pm), while others do a little longer of a fast, say 24 or 48 hours, once a month. During those fasts, you should consume plenty of water, herbal teas without sugar, and fresh juices – these allow your body to continue absorbing certain nutrients while giving your digestive system a rest. Also drinking water with a dash of salt to keep you from becoming lightheaded. Please check with your doctor before starting any diet.

There are also detox cleanses, which should be done with every change of the season. These should last 10 to 10 to 21 days – (about 3 weeks). You must seek advice and assistance from your doctor or a nutritional therapist before undertaking one of these to avoid complications while detoxing.

3. Lymphatic System

Your lymphatic system consists of your spleen, lymph nodes and lymphatic fluid. This fluid travels between your muscles as a detox waste mechanism. Your spleen is the filter of your lymphatic system. Just like a pool filter, it filters out the toxins accumulated from your lymph nodes.

When you don't exercise or drink enough water, there is no water flow or muscle contraction to force the fluid through the body, so the toxins accumulate between your muscles and in your lymphatic system. Failure to exercise or drink enough water daily, led to water retention and toxicity. If you want to lose weight this is extremely important. Toxins build up in the body daily from skin products, bad food, and our environment. You can tell if you hold on to water if at the end of the day your face, under your eyes, or your ankles and feet are puffy. These symptoms can also be connected to another spoke such as digestion. If you often feel bloated and puffy after eating food it is an indication you have difficulty digesting it.

4. Hormones

The fifth spoke on your weight loss wheel is hormones. Hormonal imbalances are common and are usually indicated by mood swings, frustration, anger, skin issues, and weight gain. One of the first indications of hormonal imbalances for women is weight gain linked to the thyroid. Pregnancy can reveal hormonal imbalances too, especially when a woman suffers from nausea, bloating, and vomiting – all of these are natural during pregnancy but are signs hormones are not balanced.

If you don't sleep well – perhaps tossing and turning all night, then wake up feeling more tired than when you went to bed, there's a good chance your hormones are very imbalanced. This too leads to weight gain.

What you eat affects how your body produces the hormone insulin. Insulin is produced in the pancreas and helps regulate your blood sugar. When you eat, your food breaks down and produces blood sugars that enter your bloodstream. This signals the pancreas to produce insulin, which helps the blood sugar enter your cells so your body can use it for energy. When blood sugar enters the cells, it comes out of your bloodstream, which signals the pancreas to reduce insulin production.

Too much sugar enters your bloodstream when you eat a diet high in sugar, processed foods, and carbohydrates. That means the pancreas must work overtime, producing more insulin to cope with demand and, your cells will stop responding to it. The pancreas pushes even more insulin out to make them respond but it simply can't keep up with demand and your blood sugar levels will continue to rise.

The human body can only burn so much energy; unused energy is stored as fat. When your blood sugar and insulin levels continue to rise, more fat is stored, thus causing weight gain. The only way to stop this from happening is through your diet. Two of the best diets are the keto diet or a plant-based diet – the more plant-based foods you can eat, the better. Keep flour, dairy, and sugar out of your diet because they are the worst three foods for weight gain.

5. Stress

The fifth spoke in our wheel is stress, and that's where the cortisol hormone comes in. Stress is a common factor in daily life, and a certain amount is good for you. It can help keep your brain tuned and improve your health and performance. Too little and you are likely to feel bored, but too much can lead to anxiety, which leads to poor health.

Many of my patients have told me they can't understand why they are not losing weight. They eat a healthy diet rich in vegetables and fruits, but their weight simply won't decrease. A deeper look told me that many of these people are bogged down by stress. Some were going through a divorce, had lost a close family member, were preparing to get married or have a baby. Not all stress is caused by negative events, but good or bad, it all takes its toll on your health.

People under stress generally don't sleep well and are depressed or anxious. These are all indicators that your cortisol levels are too high. High cortisol levels trigger the liver to release more blood sugar, which triggers insulin release – and you now know that too much insulin causes weight gain.

One way to test your cortisol levels is through a spit test, done five times daily and sent off for lab testing. You should start the day with higher cortisol levels, gradually reducing throughout the day. They should be very low by nighttime, allowing you to fall into a naturally good sleep.

Like insulin, high cortisol levels are another factor that can break your weight loss wheel.

6. Your Gut

The last spoke on our wheel is an unhealthy gut. When the gut is filled with bad bacteria and yeast, it can cause problems. Many years ago, most people believed that all yeast was bad, that we didn't need it in our bodies, and it was nothing more than a parasite. We now know some yeasts are good for the body. But when we take antibiotics, use cortisone or cortisol medications, and fill our bodies with sugar, it causes the growth of bad yeasts and bacteria. These grow so much that they can overtake the good bacteria creating a poor, acidic environment in your gut. This acidity causes the weight to pile on.

The links between gut health and weight loss have been closely studied. While we've long known that the key to losing weight is a consistent deficit in calories, the latest research shows that there may indeed be a connection between gut health and weight loss too.[41]

---

[41] Gora, Anna. "Is There a Link between Gut Health and Weight Loss?" LiveScience, November 3, 2022. https://www.livescience.com/gut-health-and-weight-loss&sa=D&source=docs&ust=1719928417730223&usg=AOvVaw2yZd0f8p59d7C2L2bxs8bw.

So could improving our digestive health help us to shed unwanted pounds?

Our metabolism is a highly complex mechanism. If you've ever embarked on a weight loss journey, you may know that it's not as straightforward as 'energy in versus energy out'. How efficient our bodies are at using calories and regulating appetite will depend on a wide range of factors. Some of them cannot be changed, like our genetic make-up or age. But others, like our gut microbiota, can be modified.

If there is a connection between gut health and weight loss, this could open new possibilities. For example, probiotics and prebiotics could be used in the fight against obesity.

Gut Hormones

The constant communication between our nervous and digestive systems is central to regulating our metabolism and appetite. Gut hormones play a critical role in this exchange of information, passing on signals of nutritional status from our gut to the brain, so the brain can interpret the body's energy needs and respond to them accordingly.

Our gastrointestinal system releases over 20 different hormones involved in maintaining energy balance. The levels of these gut hormones depend on factors including the food we eat, the state of our health, and the compounds produced by our gut bacteria. Some of these hormones will directly affect our eating behavior. According to the peer-reviewed Nutrient's Journal, the hormones cholecystokinin, peptide YY, pancreatic polypeptide, glucagon-like peptide-1, and oxyntomodulin will suppress your appetite, whereas ghrelin will make you hungrier.[42]

Gut hormones are critical to weight loss. Low-calorie diets will inevitably alter their levels to promote appetite and a less efficient metabolism, as reported in the Gastroenterology Journal.[43] That's why so many people on weight loss diets may struggle with controlling their appetite and the dreaded yo-yo effect.

Gut Microbes and Obesity

There's growing evidence that people who carry excess weight tend to have a different composition of gut microbes compared with lean individuals. According to a review published in the Nutrients Journal, gut microbiota of obese people may be less diverse and contain less of the beneficial bacterial strains.[44] What is the gut-weight connection?

Our metabolism is a highly complex mechanism. If you've ever embarked on a weight loss journey, you may know that it's not as straightforward as 'energy in versus energy out'. How efficient our bodies are at using calories and regulating appetite will depend on a wide range of factors. Some of them cannot be changed, like our genetic make-up or age. But others, like our gut microbiota, can be modified.

---

[42] Alhabeeb, Habeeb et al. "Gut Hormones in Health and Obesity: The Upcoming Role of Short Chain Fatty Acids." Nutrients vol. 13,2 481. 31 Jan. 2021, doi:10.3390/nu13020481.

[43] Jie, Zhuye, Xinlei Yu, Yinghua Liu, Lijun Sun, Peishan Chen, Qiuxia Ding, Yuan Gao, et al. "The Baseline Gut Microbiota Directs Dieting-Induced Weight Loss Trajectories." Gastroenterology 160, no. 6 (January 19, 2021): 2029–42. https://doi.org/10.1053/j.gastro.2021.01.029.

[44] Liu, Bing-Nan et al. "Gut microbiota in obesity." World journal of gastroenterology vol. 27,25 (2021): 3837-3850. doi:10.3748/wjg. v27.i25.3837.

The best environment for your gut is an alkaline one. A fiber-rich green diet is the best way to achieve this, with plenty of raw vegetables, salads, and free-range/grass-fed meats, dairy, and fish. Minimize how much meat and dairy you eat. Another way to foster the right gut bacteria is to take a high-quality probiotic supplement. The only way to keep that wheel rolling is to look after it.

Testimonial

I was born with Cerebral Palsy and felt lousy all my adult life until I met Scott. I went to see Scott, and he gave me a supplement to take. The next morning, gunk came out of my eye, and my legs loosened up. It was just phenomenal. Anytime I'm not feeling good, I go see Scott. I tell him my problem, and he corrects it. Within hours, I feel like a million bucks. Scott gives me inspiration. He is a lifesaver.
–Steve, Age 51

Tips:

- Eat a whole food diet consisting of fish, organic meats, vegetables, and fruit. If it comes in a can, a bag, or a box look at the ingredients and stay away from processed foods.
- Don't shop the aisles in the store, shop the perimeter where the whole foods are found.
- Stay away from gluten and sugar which cause inflammation and weight gain.
- Drink a gallon of water every day to keep the blood flowing and water retention down.

"You must do something hard, and beyond daily life activities to look and feel great. This is done by activating the divine powers within your unique DNA."
Scott Sommer, LAc

Scan the QR Code with your Smartphone to view message about WEIGHT LOSS.

OR follow this link: https://qrco.de/weightloss_issues

Chapter 6

Toxins, Stress,
and Detoxifying Your Life

Toxic Soup

The next category is toxicity, which is a wide-ranging subject. First, there are toxins caused by heavy metals, such as arsenic. You might be surprised to learn that while dieticians and nutritionists expound on the healthy virtues of rice, it contains high levels of arsenic, especially brown rice. Many vegetables and fruits are wrapped in plastic or have been sprayed with chemicals to ensure they maintain freshness. Even products claiming to be organic may have been sprayed with chemical pesticides.

So growing your own fruits and vegetables or shopping at your local farmer's market are always the best ways to ensure what you are eating is not infected by these pesticides. You can use a fruit and veggie wash if you can only buy food riddled with pesticides. There is a great one available through Young Living Inc. There are also silver and mercury fillings, radiation from x-rays, and 5G continually bombarding our health. Heavy metals can often be found in GMO-farmed foods and common toiletries. Unless it is organic, everything you eat has a chemical in it or on it.

Sick From the Inside Out

Diet and lifestyle can change everything if you are sick – not a bag of prescription meds your doctor told you to take.

"You try many medicines in vain, but there is no healing for you."
–Jeremiah 46:11

Medications treat symptoms while nutrition heals the body naturally. I'm not advocating quitting any drug cold turkey. I always work slowly and methodically with my patients and their doctors to gradually decrease the dosages of medications while replacing them with the natural equivalent. In some cases, certain medications are required and cannot be replaced with alternative means, but this is a very small percentage. A healthy diet and lifestyle certainly go a long way in helping your body to heal. God created herbs and plants for healing your body naturally.

"Your healing medicine will be made from the leaves of trees."
–Ezekiel 47:12

Sadly, many people don't discern when they are in trouble. Typically because most people think there are a range of symptoms that just come with aging. Many suffer from hormonal imbalances, anxiety, depression, acne, skin outbreaks, unexplained pain, constant indigestion, aching joints, headaches, cancer and auto-immune diseases, etc. My goal is to teach you the truth. These conditions are caused by poor food choices, lack of water, lack of nutrition, and sedentary lifestyles. The longer you sit back and accept these as a normal part of aging, the harder it will be.

The older you get, the more toxins there are, and the harder it is to remove them. When your body works well on the inside, you look and feel great on the outside. One of the biggest factors in this is your body's own garbage disposal system – the liver, kidneys, and spleen.

All of these systems filter your body. If you are careful and only expose yourself to minimal amounts of toxins and external forces, these natural systems of the body do their job well. Yet, sadly, we live in a world full of harmful chemicals, electrical pollution, and ultra-processed foods. The human body can only handle so much, and once you overload your system with toxins, they start to build up.

Imagine a waste disposal plant where all your rubbish is taken out and dumped. It sits there, gradually rotting away and turning into sludge. That's what happens in your body when you don't clean out the garbage. It rots inside you (constipation), often causing cell and tissue damage. The longer it sits in the body, the worse the damage gets.

It's up to us to find out how to unlock the storage units in our bodies where all the decomposing rubbish sits. The colon and excess body fat are the two most common places we store toxins. Pain, swelling, and stiffness are signals we are riddled with toxins. When toxins spread throughout the body, they irritate your nerves, causing stiff joints and a lack of energy. It takes a concentrated effort to rid the body of toxins through drinking enough water, clean eating, and detox therapies. I have invested in detox therapies from all over the world to accelerate the healing process of my patients. I have also been designing custom detox nutritional programs to take home consisting of whole food supplements, systemic formulas, and custom detox elixirs, specifically formulated for the type of toxicity.

You must invest in your health and become in tune with your body. You will then know when you are experiencing a symptom, so you can resolve it as soon as possible. Most people invest in their 401K but neglect their health then they retire and are too sick or in too much pain to enjoy it. Many of my aging patients are those who neglected their health throughout their lives, are recently retired, and are now suffering from terminal illness, or the common crippling conditions of our culture.

The good news is you can start now by embracing your health and the principles in this book. My quote to patients is, *"It's never too late until it's too late."* So, invest in your health now, because what you do in this decade will ultimately determine your next decade.

Clean-Up Time

The most effective way of healing ourselves from the inside out is to release toxins and rid them from the body. Toxins enter through our mouth, skin, and breath. In our clinic, we use therapies such as professional grade ionic detox foot baths to help our patients.[45] The foot bath is a negative ion generator which travels up through the pores of the feet through the lymphatic system and attracts the toxin which are attracted to opposite polarity (charge). Then they are pulled out through the lymphatic system the same way they came in.

We also have found that infrared saunas, the Hocatt (An oxygen-ozone therapy), Hyperthermic Heat Pods (such as the Slimwell), Firefly Light Therapy, and the Japanese E Power Belt work extremely well at killing the toxins in your body and clearing out the backlog

---

[45] Learn more here: "Optimum Detox Footbaths – Key Concepts, Benefits, Research, FAQ, Buyers Guide, Comparisons." Hymbas. Accessed July 19, 2024. https://www.hymbas.com/optimum-detox-footbath-key-concepts.php#Learn.

in your liver and kidneys. Once that backlog is cleared, they can do what they do best: clear the rest of the toxins out of your system.

Consider how these toxins got into your body. Think back to environments you may have been in when you were younger. Were you a mechanic spending your days coated in oil and grease? Were you breathing in odorous fumes from materials? Take my dad, for example. He was a painter and wall covering contractor surrounded by paint and paste all day every day. Those chemicals gradually accumulated in his body. I taught him how to remove those toxins from his body, extending his life and making him healthy again from the inside out.

Similarly, my mom was a cosmetologist and beautician, spending her days surrounded by highly noxious hair dyes and other strong chemicals. Her skin would erupt in rashes, and her hands would crack and start bleeding. I felt for her, knowing that she spent the days surrounded by substances that were damaging her body. The lesson here is to look back in your life to determine if you were exposed to toxic chemicals sometime in your own life.

What are PFA's?

Short for "per-and polyfluoroalkyl substances," PFAS are a class of thousands of man-made synthetic chemicals that have been around since the 1940s. They are found in everything from cosmetics to outdoor gear, non-stick pans, food wrappers, and countless others, according to the CDC.[46] They are forever chemicals which end up in

---

[46] "Per and Polyfluoroalkyl Substances (PFAS) and Your Health." Centers for Disease Control and Prevention, January 18, 2024. https://www.atsdr.cdc.gov/pfas/index.html.

landfills, and seep into our soil, air, and drinking water. This means that they end up in food, wildlife, and even our bloodstream.

Facts about PFAS:

- Used widely to reduce friction or resist oil, water, and stains.
- Widespread and persistent in the environment.
- Among studied PFAS: absorbed in intestines and lungs; bind to serum and tissue proteins; most not metabolized; half-lives range from a few days to 8+ years

These harmful chemicals pollute the world and never break down. Exposure to PFAS is linked to a range of health problems, especially for those that work in the manufacturing industry, or who drink contaminated water. The Agency for Toxic Substances and Disease Registry says exposure to PFAS may lead to higher risk for kidney or testicular cancer, increased cholesterol levels, as well as damage to the liver and immune system.[47] In 2016, the EPA said PFAS were not a threat at low levels: 70 parts per trillion. The agency just changed that advisory, lowering the "safe" threshold to essentially zero. PFAS still pose risks at levels so low that they're not detected, the EPA said.[48]

Keep in mind that anything that goes on your skin goes into your body, and it doesn't exit the body as quickly as it entered.

---

[47] "Pfas Information for Clinicians Factsheet." Centers for Disease Control and Prevention, January 18, 2024. https://www.atsdr.cdc.gov/pfas/resources/pfas-information-for-clinicians-factsheet.html.

[48] Ryan, Erika, Mary Louise Kelly, and Patrick Jarenwattananon. "PFAS 'Forever Chemicals' are everywhere. Here's what you should know about them.". *All Things Considered*. NPR, June 22, 2022.

Hundreds of years ago, we knew nothing of germs and bacteria. We relied on herbs and plants for medicine. Think about the early days when they didn't have processed foods; they had natural wholefood and grains, meat, fruit, fish, and plants that were safe to eat. We didn't have cars or machinery; we had horses and walking for transportation. We used our hands to make the things we needed or wanted. We used natural materials to make those things. We didn't have chemicals – we had fresh, clean air to breathe and natural spring water to drink.

We now consume GMO crops, which have been genetically modified and manipulated to produce bigger produce and vegetables. Ever notice how large some of these vegetables and fruits are in the store? Many of our health issues began with GMOs. Our stores are full of processed foods, bad fats, sugar, and salt, while fresh, organic foods are too expensive for many people to buy. This is why much of the population is sick and struggling.

Emotional Toxicity

"A tranquil mind gives life to the body, but jealousy rots the bones."
–Proverbs 14:30

We can't leave out emotional toxicity. We all know someone who is toxic abusive, dishonest, dysfunctional, or eternally negative. They cause stress in our lives. This often leads to sickness or other serious conditions, so you must guard your heart, mind, and personal space. You can pray for them and help them from a distance, but you should not spend time with them.

Emotions affect our health both positively and negatively. What we take to heart, what we choose to watch, and what we choose to listen to can also be bad for our health. Negative or hurtful words are felt in your mind, heart, and body. It is very much a part of why some people are sick. Have you ever read the study on speaking negatively to one plant, while speaking positively to another?[49] One becomes wilted, while the other blooms and thrives. Negative words can damage your health. So, choose positive people, thoughts, and words.

You must remove yourself from harmful relationships, workplaces, movies, and music, etc. These can cause physical and emotional sickness. Surround yourself with only those who challenge, inspire, and motivate you to do better and be better. You will become like the people you surround yourself with, so choose your friends carefully. Sometimes, emotional traumas and anxieties are unavoidable, but even then, you can manage it with therapy, a clean diet, exercise, herbs, and supplements. There are many natural ways to strengthen your resolve and enable you to plow through stress victoriously.

Managing Stress Through Exercise

Exercise works the body, muscles, and bones and prepares you for a stressful event. It enables you to handle stress without experiencing common physical reactions to stress, such as heart attacks, strokes, and emotional outbursts. In essence, stressing the body protects you from stress itself, both physically and mentally. So, to manage stress, you should begin exercising. Exercise also helps alleviate anxiety and depression because it releases dopamine and serotonin into the brain. These are the chemicals that make you feel good and happy.[50]

---

[49] "IKEA Conducts Bullying Experiment on Plants – the Results Are Shocking – National." Global News, May 18, 2018. https://globalnews.ca/news/4217594/ bully-a-plant-ikea/#.

[50] McGonigal, Kelly. "Five Surprising Ways Excercise Changes Your Brain." *Greater Good Magazine.* Greater Good Magazine, January 6, 2020. https://greatergood. berkeley.edu/article/item/five_surprising_ways_exercise_changes_your_brain#:~.

Many of my patients come to me dependent on anxiety medications and antidepressants and suffer from the side effects of these pharmaceutical drugs. They feel even more depressed, unable to sleep, and so on. Did you know if you start on a regular exercise regime, you can gradually wean yourself off these drugs? Our creator rewards those who are not slothful by increasing their happy hormones, giving us an A for effort.

Testimonial

I had a foot bath to remove toxins from my body. I liked how Dr. Sommer came in at the end of my detox and informed me and my husband what primarily was in the bath. We both removed many disgusting toxins from our bodies through the pores in our feet!
– Kelly Zufelt

Tips for a Whole-Body Detox:
The 90-Day Challenge

Start with the 90-day challenge to eat better. If you are accustomed to filling your body with bad foods, the first few days will be very hard, but stick with it. If you feed your body nutrient-dense foods, you will feel and see the difference as the days pass. I call it the Whole-Food Organic Diet:

- Meat (in moderation), vegetables, and fruits. Shopping the outer rim of the grocery store.
- I recommend the Blue Zone Diet.[51] Blue zones are the areas in the world with the healthiest, longest-living populations,

---

[51] "Blue Zones." Bluezones.com. Accessed July 19, 2024. https://www.bluezones.com/.

including Okinawa, Japan; Sardinia, Italy; Nicoya, Costa Rica; Ikaria, Greece; and Loma Linda, California.

- Start juicing my PLAC formula (Parsley, lemon, apple and celery) every day. I recommend a cold pressed wide feed juicer such as the Nama J2 juicer.52 Nama also sends a recipe book with their juicer. (After using many cold-pressed juicers we have found this one to be the best because it's so easy to clean). There are fantastic juicing books on Amazon as well.
- I remember as a child my grandparents juiced parsley, lemon, apple and carrots and celery daily (PLAC) and snuck it into the hospital when my mom was paralyzed from the neck down with Guillain-Barre' Syndrome. She soon recovered; I believe because of the juicing. The benefits of juicing are endless. My wife and I also try to juice pineapple, ginger and greens daily.
- When experiencing detox, drink 32 oz of water with lemon daily.

Within a week, you will start feeling much better, full of energy, and much more vibrant. Your brain fog will disappear, your memory will return, and you will be much more focused than you were before. Your skin will become more supple and glowing, and your hair will come alive. You will feel healthier on the inside and look healthier on the outside. That alone is enough to encourage you to continue the challenge; once the 90 days are up, keep pushing on. Day by day, let it become your lifestyle. You will thrive and feel alive.

When you live a clean life, your body will repay you with health and vitality. Fill your body with nutrients and clean water, and you will transform your body, your health, and your life.

---

52 Find these juicers on namawell.com

"You have two choices. Seek to understand the root cause of your symptoms and work side by side your body or drag your body along in frustration and settle for a Tylenol."
Scott Sommer, LAc

Scan the QR Code with your Smartphone to view message about:
TOXINS, STRESS AND DETOXIFYING YOUR LIFE.

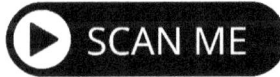

OR follow this link: https://qrco.de/toxins_stress

Chapter 7

Cellular Health

The Foundation of Our Bodies: Cellular Health

Your body is like a sports car. What you put into it is what you get out of it. If you maintain it, tune it up, change the oil, rotate the tires, and treat it responsibly, then it should last you a very long time. But if you neglect it, don't check the oil, and put the wrong fuel in the tank, you will blow the engine before you know it. Aging is something that will happen to all of us, of course.

The real choice is whether we age gracefully or faster than necessary. Aging gracefully, in my mind, is like a classic car. It's well taken care of, and it lasts longer than you would ever expect. In a parade it looks like an older car, but it is in mint condition.

The other option is not so great, like a farmer who left his car out in the field abandoned to the elements. Or, in a less extreme scenario, just someone who has a car but doesn't take care of it. The car eventually stops running and falls into disrepair. Eventually, the paint peels (the skin), and the body becomes rusted, corroded, and imperfect. Over time, it becomes completely immobile and ready for the junkyard.

This is parallel to your body over time.

Cellular health is all about how your body functions on the inside. These cells are like the car's engine and keeping you strong is all about keeping those cells healthy. The human body is made of more than 37 trillion cells. Every part of your body has different cells, but many are duplicates, and there are only so many different types. For example, the cells in your skin are the same as in your gut.

Let me tell you about one of my experiences as a practitioner of Asian medicine. One of my starting points was to help design a detox program to help people come off of harmful illicit drugs. The program was offered through the state. People sent to us would start on protein shakes and powders, followed by acupuncture, which would help calm their nervous system. Once they had begun healing from the inside, we would teach them how to improve their lifestyle. This included cooking and nutrition lessons. However, the one thing we noticed they all suffered from was poor cellular health.

How Could we Tell?

One of the biggest indicators was their teeth – visibly decaying and falling out. The drugs were rapidly aging their cells and bodies, while also damaging their gums and teeth. Their skin made them look much older than they were. It was like leather, dry and wrinkled. The difference between these people and healthy people was stunningly obvious. The healthy people looked younger than their actual age, their skin was glowing, and they looked healthy and alive – one of the first indicators of good cellular health.

The unhealthy patients suffered from digestive issues. What is in your gut is reflected in your complexion.

One symptom of inflammatory bowel disease (IBD), for example, is skin rashes or lesions. Research suggests that the connection also goes the other way: inflammatory skin diseases like psoriasis, acne, eczema, atopic dermatitis, and rosacea may stem from microbiome imbalances. In fact, studies of people with rosacea show that certain bacteria are more abundant in their gut microbiomes than in the general population. Age-related microbiome changes may affect the skin's production of moisturizing factors, creating an accelerated rate of skin aging. Information gathered from the National Center for Biotechnology found that bacterial pathways in the gut affect the body's production of ceramides and fatty acids – natural moisturizers that fortify the skin barrier, maintain elasticity, and prevent sagging.[53]

How to Tell if Your Cells Are Healthy

So, how can you tell if your cells are healthy? First, let's look at the skin. It should be supple, moist, and glowing. This happens naturally when you drink enough water, eat a clean diet, exercise, and have a healthy gut biome. Moisturizers and lotions can soften it, but moist, plump, and supple skin comes from hydration and a healthy diet.

Your eyes should be clear and sparkling, indicating a healthy lymphatic system. Eating the wrong diet, not exercising, and having an unhealthy gut will make your eyes look dull and affect your eyesight. Poor nutrition can affect the nervous system, especially eyesight. After years of a junk food diet, one 17-year-old boy developed hearing loss. Tragically, he later went blind![54] This story

---

[53] "Gut Health and Skin: How Are They Connected?" OneSkin, March 10, 2023. https://www.oneskin.co/blogs/reference-lab/gut-health-and-skin-how-are-they-connected?u.

[54] Harrison, Rhys, Vicki Warburton, Andrew Lux, and Denize Atan. "Blindness Caused by a Junk Food Diet." *Annals of Internal Medicine* 171, no. 11 (September 30, 2019): 859. https://doi.org/10.7326/l19-0361.

was a wake-up call to parents and pediatricians because it showed the effects of a poor diet on young people.

Your nails should be strong and healthy, smooth, and without ridges. Your cuticles should have moons, and your nails should grow rapidly. You shouldn't have any fungal issues with your nails, either. Asian medicine works on the principle that each nail represents an organ system in our bodies. Issues with certain toes indicate issues with a certain organ – for example, the right big toe is linked to the liver and the digestive system.

Lastly, the tongue is a big indicator of cellular health. If your tongue has a thick yellow coating, it indicates inflammation and infection somewhere in the body. Each part of your tongue, like your nails, is linked to a specific body part. The back of the tongue indicates the tonsils, while the sides indicate the liver. The coating reveals where the issue lies in your body.

We heal from the inside out, from the top down, and how healthy our cells are depending on how we live our lives.

Signs of Poor Cellular Health

- Red, puffy, or swollen eyes upon waking
- Excessive wrinkles on your face and body
- Dry skin, red, peeled, and cracked feet
- The face is puffy, swollen, or has red cheeks (rosacea)
- Legs are swollen and feel heavy
- Varicose veins, spider veins, or bulging veins
- Dry, flat, brittle hair and/or hair loss
- Nails that are brittle, splitting, or thinning

Cellular Damage

Human beings can only be as healthy as the sickest cells in their bodies. If just one tooth is bad or if just one nail gets a fungal infection, it can bring down our entire bodies.

So, what causes our cells to age faster than they should? A small part is down to genetics, while, for the most part, it's caused by epigenetics. Which is what, exactly?

Epigenetics is the study of how your behaviors and environment can cause changes that affect the way your genes work. Unlike genetic changes, epigenetic changes are reversible.[55] It can be likened to a panel of switches or electrical circuits. If some of those switches or circuits are bad, it leads to inflammation and cellular aging. Inflammation is one of the biggest markers of many serious diseases, and the less we have in our bodies, the healthier our cells are.

Some things that cause this inflammation and faster cellular aging are eternal toxins, such as radiation exposure (CT scans, X-rays, cellular phones, etc.), and environmental toxins. That's not to mention the toxins we consume in our food – preservatives, artificial coloring, artificial sweeteners, etc. None of these are safe, nor are they natural. They are nothing less than chemicals that can destroy your liver and cause premature aging. Most pharmaceutical medications, including over-the-counter painkillers such as aspirin, can cause inflammation if overused.

---

[55] "Epigenetics, Health, and Disease," Centers for Disease Control and Prevention, accessed July 22, 2024, https://www.cdc.gov/genomics-and-health/about/epigenetic-impacts-on-health.html.

Other factors that cause cellular damage include not drinking enough purified water and lack of deep sleep. The human body is a marvelous machine of interconnected systems that rely on one another and external factors to work properly. We already have a built-in waste system that eliminates toxins, but it needs help. We need water to help our bodies flush out the toxins and stop excess toxins from building up. Constantly using skin lotions and makeup that contain lead (many of them do) adds to our everyday stresses. This affects cellular health and our ability to function normally throughout the day.

Did you know that many beauty and grooming products contain lead? According to the FDA, cosmetics like eyeshadows, eyeliners, blushes, shampoos, and body lotions all contain low levels of lead.[56] Using skin lotions and makeup that contain lead affects cellular health and our ability to function normally. Hazardous ingredients like this can affect cellular health. Everything we do or don't do contributes to the health of our cells. The cleaner we live our lives, the less stress our cells are under, and the less damage will occur.

Soil to Your Body

Think of your body in terms of how trees or plants grow. The more you feed and water them with the right nutrients, the healthier they grow. I took part in an experiment in high school involving growing corn. Although all the plants were the same, they all grew differently, depending on the nutrients in the water (the blood). Some corn plants turned yellow, indicating a nitrogen deficiency, while some turned purple, indicating a lack of phosphorus. Some turned brown-

---

[56] Center for Food Safety and Applied Nutrition. "Lead in Cosmetics." U.S. Food and Drug Administration. Accessed July 19, 2024. https://www.fda.gov/cosmetics/potential-contaminants-cosmetics/lead-cosmetics#:~:text=Our%20data%20show%20that%20over,a%20maximum%20of%2010%20ppm.

black, meaning they could not produce chlorophyll, which indicated sick plants.

The Four Primary Tissue Types

The term tissue describes a group of cells that are similar in structure and perform a specific function. Learning about the primary tissue types in the human body is essential for understanding the structure and function of organs. These tissues work together to contribute to the overall health and maintenance of the human body. The body's foundation is made of 4 different combinations of tissues; they are organized into four categories: epithelial, connective, muscle, and nervous.[57]

1. **Epithelial tissue** refers to groups of cells that cover the exterior surfaces of the body, line internal cavities and passageways, and form certain glands.
2. **Connective tissue,** as its name implies, binds the cells and organs of the body together.
3. **Muscle tissue** contracts forcefully when excited, providing movement.
4. **Nervous tissue** is also excitable, allowing for the generation and propagation of electrochemical signals in the form of nerve impulses that communicate between different regions of the body.

---

[57] Biga, Lindsay M., Staci Bronson, Sierra Dawson, Amy Harwell, Robin Hopkins, Joel Kaufmann, Mike LeMaster, et al. "4.1 Types of Tissues." Anatomy Physiology, September 26, 2019. https://open.oregonstate.education/aandp/chapter/4-1-types-of-tissues/.

TYPES OF TISSUES

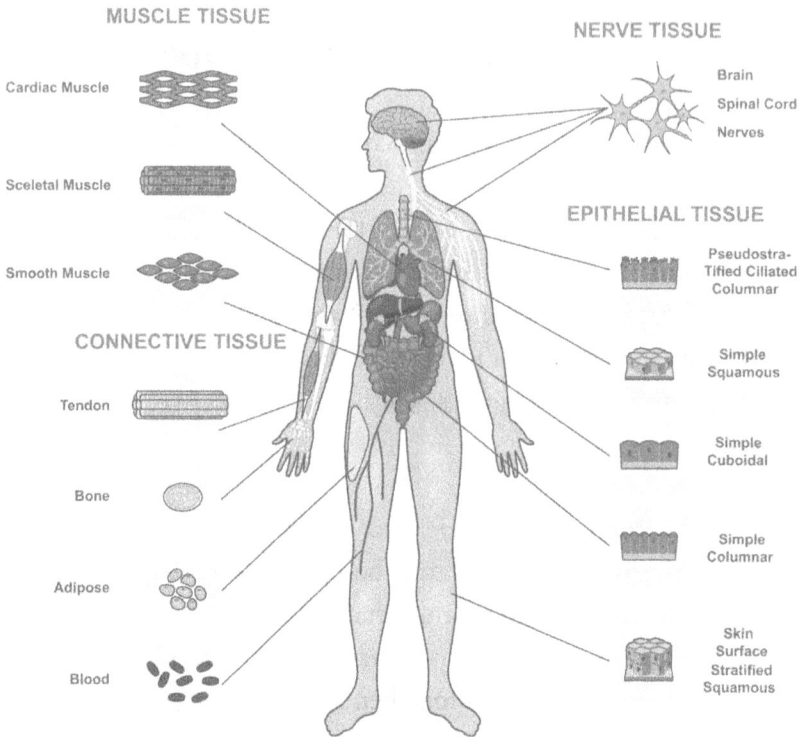

MUSCLE TISSUE

Cardiac Muscle

Sceletal Muscle

Smooth Muscle

CONNECTIVE TISSUE

Tendon

Bone

Adipose

Blood

NERVE TISSUE

Brain
Spinal Cord
Nerves

EPITHELIAL TISSUE

Pseudostra-
Tified Ciliated
Columnar

Simple
Squamous

Simple
Cuboidal

Simple
Columnar

Skin
Surface
Stratified
Squamous

Connective Tissue Membranes

A connective tissue membrane is built entirely of connective tissue. This type of membrane may be found encapsulating an organ, such as the kidney, or lining the cavity of a freely movable joint (e.g., shoulder). When lining a joint, this membrane is called a synovial membrane. Cells in the inner layer of the synovial membrane release synovial fluid. This natural lubricant enables the bones of a joint to move freely against one another with reduced friction.

Five Currently Recognized Autoimmune Connective Tissue Diseases:[58]

- **Systemic lupus erythematosus:** is an autoimmune disease involving the inability to form and the loss of self-tolerance of nuclear autoantigens and immune complexes. It causes inflammation of multiple organ systems. Due to an abnormal immune response, patients may present with widely varying serological abnormalities and symptoms that may involve the skin, joints, nervous system, lungs, kidneys, or blood vessels. This condition is more common in female and non-white individuals.
- **Scleroderma, or systemic sclerosis**: is a rare autoimmune disease that is more common in males and is characterized by autoantibodies, abnormal vascular structures, and fibrosis of the skin and various organs due to excess collagen production.
- **Myositis:** another rare autoimmune disease involving autoantibodies and variable patient presentations involving muscle tissue inflammation.
- **Rheumatoid arthritis (RA):** is an autoimmune connective tissue disease that results in chronic inflammation of body tissues, typically the joints, and may result in disability.
- **Sjogren syndrome** is a rare autoimmune disease characterized by dry eyes and mouth and damage to other organ systems such as the liver, lungs, kidneys, and central nervous system.

---

[58] Kamrani, Payvand, Geoffrey Marston, Taflin C. Arbor, and Arif Jan. "Anatomy, Connective Tissue." StatPearls [Internet]., March 5, 2023. https://www.ncbi.nlm.nih.gov/books/NBK538534/#.

Muscle Tissue

Individual muscle cells are grouped to form a fiber. These fibers bundle together to form a fascicle, and fascicles combine to create the entire muscle. Connective tissue exists between every muscle cell, fiber, and fascicle. All peripheral nerve fibers consist of three connective tissue layers, which serve as a protective connective sheath. Collagen and elastin compose the dry mass of tendon connective tissue.[59] Tendons are connective tissue structures comprised of a hierarchical arrangement of collagen molecules that arrange into collagen fibrils and then collagen fibers. Collagen fibers are organized into primary, secondary, and tertiary bundles. The tendon is surrounded by the epitenon (a fine connective tissue sheath). The complex multidimensional arrangement of the collagen fibers of tendons makes their function possible even when longitudinal, rotational, and transverse forces are exerted upon tendons.

Finding the Volcano

When you think of inflammation, what comes to mind? To many people, that word produces images of redness, swelling, heat, and pain. While you can see some types of minor inflammation, such as an infected cut on your hand or a mosquito bite, the worst types of inflammation are invisible. But what, what is inflammation?

Usually, inflammation is a natural occurrence in your body when your white blood cells jump into action to protect you from viral and bacterial attackers. Think about it. You don't feel too well when you get a chest infection, and you cough up mucus. When your

---

[59] Kamrani, Payvand, Geoffrey Marston, Taflin C. Arbor, and Arif Jan. "Anatomy, Connective Tissue." StatPearls [Internet]., March 5, 2023. https://www.ncbi.nlm.nih.gov/books/NBK538534/#.

body is fighting off invading forces, the natural reaction is known as acute inflammation. Uncomfortable as it may be, it usually goes away within hours or a few days.

However, sometimes, your immune system will trigger inflammation when there is nothing to fight against. It sees your regular body tissues and cells as unhealthy and diseased, even when they are not, and attacks them. This causes long-term damage and can lead to serious diseases. This is known as chronic inflammation and can lead to type 2 diabetes, cancer, heart disease, strokes, and much more.

The symptoms of inflammation vary widely, depending on what has caused it.

Some of the symptoms to look for are:

- stuffy or runny nose
- red eyes
- fungal infections
- varicose veins
- swollen tongue
- excess belly fat
- bloating
- general aches and pains; or
- constant coughs and colds

We can liken this inflammation to a volcano. Why? Because it always starts in one place, and it has the potential to erupt into something so much more. Let me illustrate this with a skin condition I see commonly in my patients. Skin eruptions can be cured with pills and lotions, but if it happens constantly, it could be inflammation. Somewhere in your body, there is a volcano making itself known by continually causing rashes and spots on your skin. By treating the eruption, you only treat the symptoms when you need to treat the cause.

One of the most common places where inflammation starts is the gut or digestive system. Most of us have heard of leaky gut syndrome, which is the lava flow from your volcano. The lava flows out of your gut and into the rest of your body. It can go anywhere, but usually, it will head for one of your filtration organs – kidneys, liver, spleen, etc. Getting rid of the volcano requires you to find it, which means following the lava trail right back to where it started. You also need to find what causes your volcano to erupt. For some, it is sugar; for others, it might be excess carbohydrates, too much fat, tobacco, alcohol, etc. Once you discover your tipping point, you must eliminate it. Otherwise, the volcano will continue erupting, leading to more permanent damage and long-term diseases.

However, extinguishing the volcano and stopping the lava flow doesn't mean your body will be healed immediately. Years of damage take time to heal, and if you fall back into your old ways, that volcano will reignite and start spewing lava back into your system. Next, let's look at what can go wrong in our blood.

Blood Disorders and Traditional Chinese Medicine (TCM)

The human body is like a plant or tree – it needs air, soil, water, and sun. In Asian medicine, blood is the mother of Chi (the cells' energy, mainly the mitochondria.)

TCM has a different perspective on blood compared to Western Medicine. In Western Medicine, blood is looked at through its components: red blood cells, white blood cells, platelets, and plasma.

TCM views the state of blood in the body holistically; it looks at someone's general vitality, pulse, signs of paleness (face, tongue, nails), and even the menstrual cycle. Blood nourishes our muscles, tendons, and ligaments, moistens our skin and hair, and roots our Spirit. Different factors can affect the building of blood: digestive weakness, overexercise, overwork, stress, genetics, and diet. Women are especially vulnerable to blood deficiency due to the monthly menstrual cycle, as well as blood loss from labor and childbirth. I will break down the symptoms of blood deficiency and then offer some diet and lifestyle advice to help nourish your blood.

Signs of Blood Deficiency

TCM categorizes blood deficiency into three main types. Here are the types, and the signs of blood deficiency:

Liver Blood Deficiency	Heart Blood Deficiency	Spleen Blood Deficiency
Amenorrhea (Scant or missing menstrual bleeding)	Insomnia	Fatigue
Cramping pain, tingling, or numbness of the limbs, shoulder, or back.	Anxiety and heart palpitations	Pale face and lips
Insomnia and sleep disturbances	Pale face	Low appetite
Dry hair, brittle nails	Poor Memory and fatigue	Weak muscles
Blurred vision or floaters in the eyes	Dizziness	Loose stools

Iron levels are crucial to blood and good mental health. Iron helps red blood cells perform the critical function of ferrying oxygen around the body. According to the University of Michigan, iron "helps your body make the molecules that are needed to make key brain chemicals... serotonin, dopamine, and norepinephrine."[60] In fact, iron deficiencies have been linked to depression and anxiety. If you drink coffee with meals, you reduce iron absorption by around 39%. For tea, that number jumps to 64%.[61]

The blood's function is known as cellular exchange – it delivers nutrients to the cells and removes waste from them. Like a UPS driver, it delivers the goods but also picks up the waste. Things start falling apart when circulation and nutrients are deficient. The blood can't deliver the goods. It's stagnant; this is called blood stagnation and blood deficiency. Stagnant circulation is the cause of many diseases. Your blood doesn't move, so it is toxic and thick.

Change how you feed the soil by changing your lifestyle, and you change how the plant (your body) grows.

Testimonial

Prior to holistic treatments, Dennis was on daily high blood pressure medicine, cholesterol medicine, medication to lower his uric acid levels, and anti-acid medication for his stomach. His blood pressure was 190/90, he was prediabetic, his kidneys and liver were showing signs of failure, and he had painful gout limiting his movement. He had a colonoscopy in

---

[60] "Could Low Iron Be Making Your Mental Health Symptoms Worse?: Psychiatry: Michigan Medicine." Michigan Medicine, June 2, 2023. https://medicine.umich.edu/dept/psychiatry/news/archive/202305/could-low-iron-be-making-your-mental-health-symptoms-worse.

[61] Morck, T A et al. "Inhibition of food iron absorption by coffee." *The American journal of clinical nutrition* vol. 37,3 (1983): 416-20. doi:10.1093/ajcn/37.3.416.

2016 in which several golf-ball-sized polyps were removed. He was put on a schedule for a colonoscopy every 3 years.

After food poisoning, Dennis was prescribed strong antibiotics, which resulted in C-diff. Dennis lost over 50 pounds due to constant nausea, stomach acid, and intestinal pain. Dennis had nodules on his thyroid, which were large enough to change his voice. He was prescribed medication that would destroy his thyroid.

In 2021, Dennis sought treatment from Scott and was given a program of specific foods to eat and to avoid, a regime of supplements, and a routine of regular weekly footbaths.

Today (2024), a scan revealed no nodules on his thyroid, and a recent colonoscopy was clean; in fact, the doctor went through his system three (3) times because he could not believe what he was seeing. At 65 years old, Dennis is taking no traditional Western medications. His blood pressure and cholesterol are lower than they have ever been (blood pressure now 130/70), and his kidneys and liver are strong. It was a miracle!

Thank you all!
–Dennis, age 65

Tips on How to Nourish Blood

Minimize or avoid these things:	Do these things to nourish your blood:
Sugar: a little honey, maple syrup, or unrefined cane sugar is fine. Read labels because sugar is added to almost everything!	**Improving digestion:** is crucial to making healthy blood. If there are any digestive issues, they need to be resolved.
Coffee: is warming and drying. As a stimulant, it takes energy from the body without returning it.	**Eat enough:** Your body needs nutrients and food to make blood. If you are not hungry in the mornings, this is a sign of digestive weakness.
Overexercise: depletes our *qi* (vital energy) and blood. We should not feel exhausted from workouts or have chronic tendon, ligament, or muscle injuries. This will be different for everyone; listening to your body is important.	**Get the proper amount of vitamins and minerals:** iron, folic acid, and B12 are essential in the diet. To absorb iron, you need adequate vitamin C (found in bell peppers, tomatoes, kale, strawberries, oranges, kiwi, lemon juice, lime juice, thyme, and parsley).
Overwork: also depletes our *qi* (vital energy) and blood.	**Eat fermented foods:** such as kefir, sauerkraut, kimchee, kombucha, unsweetened yogurt, and true sourdough bread help with iron absorption.

Excess sweating: this could be from saunas, hot yoga, or exercise. Sweat comes from our fluids, which are required to produce blood.	**If you are vegetarian or vegan, make sure you get enough B12** in your diet. These diets are more prone to blood deficiency.
Tobacco: is very drying, toxic, and damaging to the blood.	**Avoid packaged foods:** They lack vitamins, minerals, and enzymes and often contain chemicals, dyes, and food preservatives that our bodies don't require.
Overeating or eating too many heavy foods: Eat until about 70% full.	**Eat foods that nourish the blood** (see list below)

A Helpful Guide to Foods that Nourish Blood

This list is incomplete; many more foods nourish blood than what is listed below. If you can, always choose organic foods.

Fruits:
- Grapes, apples, cherries, dates, raisins, apricots (fresh and dried), raspberries, figs, black currants, pomegranates, goji berries, plums, and avocado (in small amounts).

Vegetables:
- Beets, dark leafy greens (Swiss chard, kale, collard green, etc.), leeks, chives, spinach, carrots, seaweed, red cabbage, Brussel sprouts, potatoes, sweet potatoes, yams, artichokes,

dandelion leaf, and watercress. Squash (such as pumpkins, butternut, kabocha, spaghetti and acorn).

Organic Meat and Proteins:
- Small portions of organic meat (especially red meat), bone marrow, and liver.
- Eggs and bone broths.

Organic Grains:
- Quinoa, spelt, millet, barley, wheat (specifically ancient grains), organic corn, rice, and sweet rice.

Organic Legumes:
- Lentils, soybeans (tofu), black beans, chickpeas, aduki beans, kidney beans, fava beans, and peas.

Nuts and Seeds:
- Black and white sesame seeds, almonds, chia, pumpkin.

Mushrooms:
- Shiitake, reishi, cremini, oyster.

Molasses:
- Dissolve 1 Tbsp in hot water and drink daily.

Tea:
- Nettle, raspberry leaf, dang gui, dandelion root, and goji berry.

The Trendy Way to Live

In recent years, more and more people have begun to evaluate their lifestyle choices and how they affect their health. Improving cellular health is now one of the latest trends and one of the best you can choose to follow. You might think this is just another gimmick, but ignoring cellular health can seriously affect your health and wellness.

The most important takeaway is to be aware of your body and listen to what it tells you. Preventing disease or helping recover from it can only be done by knowing where it started, and it is all done from the inside out.

Look after your cellular health, build a strong, healthy foundation, and the rest of your body will repay you by being strong and healthy. Your life choices dictate your cellular health. If you persist in feeding your body unhealthy trans fats and fast foods full of chemicals, you will pay the price.

"It still takes sixty to ninety days to grow a tomato.
This is how the natural healing process works.
You cannot push it along.
We can only encourage the natural healing process of the body."
Scott Sommer, LAc

Scan the QR Code with your Smartphone
to view message about: CELLULAR HEALTH

OR follow this link: https://qrco.de/cellular_health

Chapter 8

Hormones

All men and women have hormones and are affected by them. When your hormones are out of balance, a whole chain of physical symptoms can follow. Weight gain, anxiety, mood swings, insomnia, fatigue, brain fog, hot flashes, low libido, and much more.

Think about this scenario: You are talking to two people. One is calm, rational, and a joy to talk to, while the other is up and down, snappy, and – quite frankly – unpleasant to be around. The first person is most likely hormonally balanced, while the second most likely is not. Here are two more examples that illustrate how both men and women are affected by hormones.

Jack, a former patient of mine, was a healthy, athletic man who worked out and skied regularly. But, as time passed, he began to slow down. He got tired, gained weight, and could not get rid of that stubborn belly fat. It all pointed to one thing – not a natural aging process, but a hormonal imbalance.

Estrogen, insulin, and cortisol cause belly fat. He couldn't understand why he was gaining weight, had suddenly lost interest in his life, and was always tired. At night, he only wanted to eat sugary foods, something he had never done before. His muscle mass was declining. When he came to me, I ran a series of tests. First, we had to rebalance his thyroid.

Then, we worked on regulating his blood sugar using supplements and changing his diet. Gradually, his energy resurfaced, and that stubborn belly fat diminished. Now in his 70s, Jack is back to exercising, skiing, and more. He told me that he was excited to wake up each day and couldn't wait to live life to its fullest. He realizes now that if he doesn't keep his hormones in balance, he'll just slide back down that slippery slope.

Now, let's talk about Jill, who was in her early 50s and suffering from awful menopause symptoms. She still has so much life to live, but she had difficulty figuring out how to make her way through her hormonal changes. She, too, had piled on the weight and couldn't lose it. She had continual night sweats and had to keep a fan on all night. Her excessive sweating led to soaked sheets and a terrible night's sleep. Her mood was off, and she was constantly irritable, which began to come between her and her family, as she also suffered from bouts of depression and anxiety. These are all common symptoms for menopausal women, but it doesn't mean you have to hopelessly suffer from them.

Jill was desperate to find a solution when she came to see me. Her hormones are back in balance thanks to food, whole food supplements, detox, mindset, and lifestyle changes. She's joyful, her night sweats and irritability are gone, the weight is coming off, her skin is better, her hair has stopped falling out and is thicker, and she feels young again.

Doctors often prescribe estrogen and progesterone replacement creams to help ease menopausal discomforts. Yet, these, too, can create many problems. Your physician may tell you that all women go through this, and you must accept it. That's not true, as these stories illustrate that getting things back in balance is critical to living a vibrant life.

Understanding why you struggle so much with hormones requires understanding what they are and how they work. In Chinese medicine, a woman's hormones change every seven years. The first change comes at age 7, then at 14, when many girls begin their periods.[62] At 21, they change again, continuing this seven-year life cycle. Men's hormones change slower than women's, usually on an eight-year cycle.

TCM 7-Year Cycle for Women[63]

Age	Stage Description
7 years	The time to build a strong foundation. She will have abundant kidney Qi for the growth of permanent teeth and body hair.
14 years	A right of passage for young women. She starts to menstruate and can conceive.
21 years	This is the step into womanhood. The kidney Qi level peaks, body development stops, and wisdom teeth grow.
28 years	Full maturity and peak physicality. She has strong muscles and bones, and thick, lustrous hair.

62 Aleisha Anderson, "Women's 7 Year Cycles," mke mindbody wellness, June 9, 2022, https://www.mkewellness.com/blog/2022/6/8/womens-7-year-cycles.

63 Dewhurst, Andrea. "The Seven Year Cycle." Period Acupuncturist, December 31, 2021. https://www.theperiodacupuncturist.co.uk/post/the-seven-year-cycle.

35 years	This phase is about self-reflection. Women may see the initial signs of aging (sallow face, wrinkles, or hair loss).
42 years	Women prepare for menopause. The three Yang meridians in the upper body begin to decline, which may lead to some facial puffiness (spleen deficiency) or dark circles under the eyes (blood stagnation).
49 years	This is the second spring or water phase in Chinese medicine. Menopause occurs, and the body goes through hormonal changes.
56 years	Rebirth and a time to celebrate.

TCM 8-Year Cycle for Men[64]

Age	Stage Description
8 years	Boys go through many developmental changes during this time. The kidney Qi consolidates, allowing for permanent teeth and body hair.
16 years	This is a vital age for men. Kidney Qi is abundant; as a result, kidney essence will transform into sperm.

---

[64] Dr. Lana Moshkovich, "The Natural Aging Process through TCM," The Natural Aging Process through TCM: Lana Moshkovich, DACM, L.AC: Chinese Medicine, 2024, https://www.nirvananaturopathics.com/blog/the-natural-aging-process-through-tcm#:~:text=TCM%20follows%20an%208%20year,at%20the%20age%20of%208.

24 years	Men's body development stops at this age and the limbs are strong. The kidney Qi level peaks, and the wisdom teeth continue to grow.
32 years	This phase is when the body reaches its peak. Men have sturdy, powerful bones and tendons.
40 years	The kidneys start to decline, leading to hair loss or loose teeth.
48 years	The body starts to show signs of aging. As the Yang-Qi starts depleting from the upper body, the face will start sagging, and hair will start graying.
56 years	The liver degenerates, leading to joint problems; kidney degeneration leads to a lower amount of essence, so vitality greatly wanes.

This is the typical progression with age, yet many defy the odds when they stay on the offense by eating clean and exercising to stay strong. Doing these things will help control the natural reduction of your hormones.

So, what makes our hormones change? Well, one thing that affects them is diet. One of my patients was a nine-year-old girl. Her first hormone change had come and gone, and she was suffering. She was irritable and emotional, often crying for no reason. Her parents didn't know how to help her, but I did. We started with herbal supplements to help balance her hormones, and then we worked on her diet. She was eating a lot of dairy and chicken, two of the worst foods for hormonal imbalance. Why? Aren't they supposed to be healthy? As stated earlier in the food chapter, most animals raised commercially are pumped full of hormones, which make their way into the cheese, milk, cream, yogurt, and meat produced by those animals. Growth hormones don't interact well with your body's natural hormones; they cause everything to go haywire.

Now, this girl is doing great. Her hormones are back in balance, and she's the happy-go-lucky child she should be, not battling hormone problems. Junk food also plays a huge part in hormonal imbalance, as does the amount of food you eat and how often you eat throughout the day.[65] The holiday season is one of the worst times, often kick-starting a cycle of consuming too much food way more than the human body needs to survive. You don't need to – eat several times a day; your body will not starve if you cut out a meal or two. In fact, it will likely thank you for it in other ways.

Think about how many meals you eat a day. Then think about what you eat. How much of it is healthy food? How much of it is necessary? Do you need to eat that much, or is it just because it's there? Overeating and emotional eating are linked to hormonal imbalances.

Hormones and Depression

Hormones have an impact on mental health. Rather than determining the root cause of the depression, some doctors will just prescribe antidepressants, which wreak havoc on your body and hormones.[66] Did you know that between 2015 and 2018, over 13% of adults over

---

[65] Nunez, Kirsten. "3 Foods (and 2 Drinks) That Can Mess with Your Hormones." Edited by Haley Mades. Real Simple, January 11, 2024. https://www.realsimple.com/worst-foods-for-hormone-health-7558543.

[66] Pavlidi, Pavlina et al. "Antidepressants' effects on testosterone and estrogens: What do we know?." *European journal of pharmacology* vol. 899 (2021): 173998. doi:10.1016/j.ejphar.2021.173998.

18 had used antidepressants recently?[67] Some forms of depression can be treated with lifestyle changes, and without the use of hormones and antidepressants.

We also know that plastic impacts the way our bodies produce hormones. Long-term exposure to plastic particles and associated chemicals has been shown to exhaust thyroid endocrine function.[68] This means the plastic in water bottles could be throwing your hormones off. The best thing to do is to avoid it as much as you can or just buy a water-purifying product like Pure Aqua Mins to add to your water. We sell this in our clinic, and you can order it online.

These are the nine major hormones that we need to keep balanced:

1. **Testosterone** is one of the principal androgens present in the body. Androgens are hormones associated with male reproduction. However, women also produce testosterone and other androgens in the ovaries, adrenal glands, and fat cells. This hormone contributes to sex drive, fat distribution, muscle strength, bone mass, and red blood cell production in both men and women. Women who have too much testosterone may have thinning hair on their heads, excess body hair, facial hair, acne, more body fat, low libido, and smaller breasts. Having high testosterone can also cause irregular periods and contribute to fertility problems.

---

[67] Brody DJ, Gu Q. Antidepressant use among adults: United States, 2015–2018. NCHS Data Brief, no 377. Hyattsville, MD: National Center for Health Statistics. 2020.

[68] Ullah, Sana et al. "A review of the endocrine disrupting effects of micro and nano plastic and their associated chemicals in mammals." *Frontiers in endocrinology* vol. 13 1084236. 16 Jan. 2023, doi:10.3389/fendo.2022.1084236.

2. **Cortisol** is a type of hormone known as a steroid hormone and is produced by the adrenal glands. It has many responsibilities that keep you healthy and energetic. Cortisol is responsible for helping regulate metabolism, regulating blood pressure, acting as an anti-inflammatory, and even forming memories. Cortisol is called a stress hormone because the body is stressed it secretes higher levels of the hormone.

    Having too much cortisol for extended periods can cause hypertension, anxiety, sleep loss, and autoimmune problems. Too little cortisol is associated with low blood pressure, weakness, and fatigue. Lack of sleep raises cortisol levels, and cortisol cranks up your blood sugar... which then plunges, making you stressed and craving junk food. Sleep affects our hormones, good or bad. When you sleep, levels of a hunger-related hormone called leptin surge, signaling to your body that you don't need to eat. If you sleep poorly, your body won't produce the right amount of leptin – so you'll feel extra hungry the next day and be more prone to weight gain.

3. **Insulin** is a hormone produced by the pancreas. It has many functions, but its main responsibility is converting glucose (sugar) in the things we eat into a form the body can use for energy. Insulin helps regulate blood sugar. When the body cannot produce or process insulin correctly, it can result in insulin resistance, prediabetes, or diabetes.

4. **Progesterone** is another hormone associated with the female reproductive system is progesterone. Like estrogen, progesterone plays a key part in the menstrual cycle. It helps prepare the uterus for pregnancy and is an important factor in the early stages of pregnancy. Low progesterone levels can cause heavy and irregular menstrual periods, as well as fertility problems.

If progesterone levels drop during pregnancy, it can cause premature labor or miscarriage. Having too much progesterone may be associated with an increased risk of breast cancer.

5. **Estrogen** is one of the key female sex hormones, but men have estrogen too. In women, estrogen is produced in the ovaries and is responsible for functions like ovulation, menstruation, breast development, and increasing bone and cartilage density. Having too much estrogen can increase the risk of certain cancers and is linked to symptoms like depression, weight gain, difficulty sleeping, headaches, low sex drive, anxiety, and menstrual problems. Having too little estrogen can cause weakened bones (osteoporosis), menstrual problems, fertility issues, and mood disorders. While estrogen levels naturally decrease with age until menopause, some conditions may cause low estrogen in women who are not yet perimenopausal.

6. **Human Growth Hormone** is often referred to by the initials HGH. Sometimes it is simply called "growth hormone." It is a type of hormone produced by the pituitary gland. As the name implies, HGH is mostly associated with growth and development. It stimulates cell growth, cell regeneration, and cell reproduction in children.

7. **Adrenaline,** like cortisol, adrenaline is known as a stress hormone. It is produced in the adrenal glands and within some cells of the central nervous system. Adrenaline's major function is to prepare the body for its "fight or flight" response and allows for quick decision making in dangerous or stressful situations. Having too much adrenaline for extended periods can lead to high blood pressure, rapid heartbeat, anxiety, heart palpitations, irritability, and dizziness.

8. **Thyroid Hormones** are produced in the thyroid gland. They perform a variety of crucial tasks in the body. One of the biggest responsibilities of the thyroid hormones is regulating metabolism. An imbalance of thyroid hormones can be linked to a serious condition like Grave's disease or Hashimoto's disease, which can cause problems with weight management and energy levels. Iodine is very important for thyroid function. Iodine is one of the most important minerals we should get from our food.[69] Without it, the thyroid cannot function as it should.

9. **Melatonin** is generated by the pineal gland. Melatonin levels peak during the nighttime hours, inducing physiological changes that promote sleep, such as decreased body temperature and respiration rate.[70] During the day, melatonin levels are low because large amounts of light are detected by the retina. Light inhibition of melatonin production is central to stimulating wakefulness in the morning and to maintaining alertness throughout the day.

Signs of Hormone Imbalances

We can start with the brain and its hormone-producing glands, like the pituitary gland. Do you get migraines or headaches? One-sided headaches? That's the pituitary gland, and it doesn't just cause headaches when it isn't working right. It can also lead to irritability, mood swings, weight gain, and problems sleeping.

The adrenal glands are tucked away at the top of your kidneys and are related to energy and cortisol. So, if you wake up feeling tired

---

[69] "How 8 Types of Hormones Affect Your Health." Kernodle Clinic, June 25, 2020. https://www.kernodle.com/obgyn_blog/how-types-of-hormones-affect-your-health/.

[70] "Melatonin." In *Encyclopedia Britannica*. Encyclopedia Britannica. Accessed July 19, 2024. https://www.britannica.com/science/melatonin.

or your energy dips throughout the day, these glands are likely not producing the right levels of hormones. How often do you feel you've run out of energy during the day? Or do you feel tired and depressed all the time? That's what hormonal imbalance does. Here is a long list of symptoms you may be suffering from to help you understand.

Common Hormone Imbalance Symptoms:

- weight gain[71]
- a hump of fat between the shoulders
- unexplained and sometimes sudden weight loss
- fatigue
- muscle weakness
- muscle aches, tenderness, and stiffness
- pain, stiffness, or swelling in your joints
- increased or decreased heart rate
- sweating
- increased sensitivity to cold or heat
- constipation or more frequent bowel movements
- frequent urination
- increased thirst
- increased hunger
- decreased sex drive
- depression
- nervousness, anxiety, or irritability
- blurred vision
- infertility
- thinning hair or fine, brittle hair
- dry skin

---

[71] O'Keefe Osborn, Corinne. "Everything You Need to Know about Hormonal Imbalance." Edited by Marina Basina. Healthline, February 9, 2023. https://www. healthline.com/health/hormonal-imbalance#signs-or-symptoms.

- puffy face
- rounded face
- purple or pink stretch marks

Fixing your Thyroid with Food

Food doesn't just feed your body with energy. The right foods and good fats *(good fats are the most important nutrients when feeding your hormones, and one of the reasons I do not recommend a vegetarian diet)*. Good foods and good fats also provide many of the important minerals and vitamins your body needs, which play a *key* role in keeping your hormones balanced. Many years ago, the soil provided the necessary nutrients to keep your hormones balanced, but now it is very challenging to get those nutrients from our food.

As I mentioned earlier, chemical fertilizers and pesticides have impacted the nutrition of our food and taken their toll on our health. That is why patients come to me to resolve these nutritional deficiencies. Understanding the necessity of whole food supplements and minerals, glandular support, herbal formulas, good fats, a low-carb diet, and exercise is extremely important.

Across the world, there are blue zones, places where people live much healthier and longer lives. These places in the world still follow healthy, chemical-free farming and eat a plant-based diet. They have the most centenarians, and they do not typically suffer from hormonal imbalances. When you eat the right diet and keep hydrated with sufficient water, your hormones will stay balanced, the hypothalamus and pituitary gland will communicate with your thyroid, and your thyroid is the key to your health and moods. An imbalanced thyroid can cause depression, sleep difficulties, weight gain, cold feelings, and irritability.

Many doctors treat thyroid problems with medication, which is, often unnecessary. When a medication isn't working, they increase it, creating even more complications. Women come to me all the time because their thyroid medication is wreaking havoc in their lives. Your diet, supplements, lifestyle, and exercise are the best ways to fix thyroid problems.

The 5 Pillars of Balanced Hormones

1. Mindset
2. Food
3. Wholefood supplements
4. Detox therapies
5. Lifestyle (namely exercise)

When you make the necessary changes above it is possible to keep these hormones balanced.

So, let me ask you this. Are you reading this because you have some of these symptoms? Are you looking for a quick fix? The bad news is that there is no quick fix, but the good news is you *can* fix them.

Testimonial

I started seeing Scott and his team in 2023 consistently when I was diagnosed with lung cancer. He helped me gather a treatment plan before and after my surgery for stage 1 lung cancer. I would not have been able to recover as well as I did without his treatment plan. I am also a huge skeptic when it comes to supplements, but they are not just your average supplements. They are food and medicine to your body that he tailors for everyone. After my lung surgery, my hormones were out of balance, and

he was able to give me supplements that put my body back in balance. I trust Scott, and now my children will see him as well. He is currently correcting my 11-year-old daughter's scoliosis [sic]. We are so blessed to have found him. Thank God for him every day.
–Veronica Lopez-Galu

These chemical messengers buzzing around inside you pretty much rule your entire system, influencing your appetite, weight, sex drive, cycle, and more. But hormonal weirdness isn't just a random occurrence over which you have no control. Certain behaviors can cause them to surge or sink – and do a number on your body in the process. Check out these nine habits that can screw up your hormones and alter your mental and physical health.

Tips to Help Balance Hormones:

1. **Sleep well and protect your sleep:** Aim for at least 8 hours of sleep a night. Make your room cold and dark and use a white noise machine or air filter to help you get a good night's rest.

2. **Stop eating 3-4 hours before bed to avoid an insulin spike**: I suggest a protein snack such as a few almonds, a small protein shake, or even one egg before bed. This will help keep you asleep and help you feel rested in the morning.

3. **Move your body daily:** Whether it's walking, dancing, swimming, or taking the stairs instead of the elevator, make sure you move daily. Resistance and/or weight training can help maintain your muscles and stabilize your metabolism. Weightlifting (even small weights) is great for strength, balance, and bone health. Movement also helps reduce stress hormones such as adrenaline.

4. **Hydrate:** Water can help decrease the symptoms of perimenopause and menopause. It should always be your primary liquid. Think about drinking throughout the day – always keep a water bottle nearby.

5. **Lower your stress hormones:** Deep breathing, stretching, relaxing with a good book, getting out into nature, enjoying a hot tub, or doing something creative that you love— singing, dancing, painting, playing a musical instrument— are all fantastic ways to relax and minimize stress.

6. **Lower body fat:** Extra body fat works against hormone balance. According to Baylor College of Medicine, a healthy body fat range is 25-31% for women and 18-24% for men, depending on age and athletic status.[72] I encourage my patients to eat a high-fiber, whole-food diet that limits ultra-processed foods. Aim to eat high-quality and high-protein foods (75 grams or more per day based on sex and activity level).

7. **Reduce or avoid stress (especially at night):** Worry and anxiety at night may lead to spiked cortisol levels, late-night stress eating, and insomnia. Cortisol Is your body's natural way of waking you up in the morning, but it should drop off at night when natural melatonin kicks in to put you to sleep.

8. **Start taking Maca:** Maca is a plant that originated in the Peruvian Andes mountains. It is a natural remedy that can be used to treat certain health issues, including infertility, low sex drive, and hormone imbalance. Some populations in Peru have trusted maca for thousands of years as food and medicine. I recommend organically sourced powdered

[72] Barnes, Taylor. "Body Fat Percentage vs. BMI – Which Is Important?" Baylor College of Medicine. Accessed July 19, 2024. https://www.bcm.edu/news/body-fat-percentage-vs-bmi-which-is-important.

maca root. Add 1-2 tsp to a smoothie or soup. It is suitable for both men and women.

9. **Start using a Rebounder:** I recommend using a Trampoline or rebounder for 5-15 minutes a day to aid hormone balance. This also reduces fatigue and menstrual discomfort, helps with weight loss, and lowers stress. Rebounding detoxifies excess hormones and toxins, which is key to a healthy endocrine system.

10. **Avoid plastic water bottles and food containers:** They disrupt hormones and are known as endocrine-disrupting chemicals, (EDC's).

Imagine a wheel with all its spokes intact. When your hormones are out of balance, one or more of those spokes are broken, and you need to find the break. Then, you can get yourself back on track. Fixing it may take time, but once you discover the right solution and make the necessary changes in your diet, you will see improvement. You may also benefit from additional herbal therapy. Herbal therapy is one of the more popular ways to balance hormones in place of pharmaceutical medication.

For example, there is some evidence that ashwagandha can help regulate stress levels and cortisol.[73] This one herb alone can help rebalance cortisol levels, improving sleep quality. Maca, as mentioned earlier in this chapter, is another herb gaining popularity as a hormone balancer for both men and women.

As mentioned before, reducing your carb intake can help regulate your blood sugar and insulin levels. Start exercising. Do a little weight

---

[73] "Office of Dietary Supplements – Ashwagandha: Is It Helpful for Stress, Anxiety, or Sleep?" NIH Office of Dietary Supplements. Accessed July 19, 2024. https://ods.od.nih.gov/factsheets/Ashwagandha-HealthProfessional/.

or resistance training. Exercising 2 or 3 times a week for just 15 to 20 minutes can stretch and build muscle. Muscle mass is incredibly important in balancing hormones. Do some aerobic activities every day to keep your mind, body, and liver healthy. Your liver function also plays an important role in hormonal balance, so start every day with half a lemon squeezed into a 32 oz glass of Himalayan salt water. The weight will fall off, the bloating will disappear, your skin will clear up, and your energy levels will rise. You'll feel as great as you did when you were younger. And who doesn't want that?

"What is aging you ask? The slow or fast degeneration of our cells, tissues and organs, muscles and bones. We can't stop it, but we can pump the brakes… naturally following ancient principles."
Scott Sommer, LAc

Scan the QR Code with your Smartphone to view message about: HORMONES

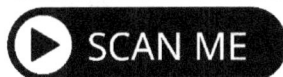

Or follow this link: https://qrco.de/our_hormones

Chapter 9

The Body Is Electric

When I was studying at UC Davis, I decided to switch from engineering to medicine to fulfill my promise to God at 9 years old. I needed to understand the human body to help people recover from brain illnesses and to prevent disease. At the time, I felt this was the only way to practice medicine: to become an MD within a Western medicine hospital or have my own practice and use natural medicine within that profession. Then, shortly before taking the MCAT, I read a book in the library. This book was about Asian Medicine, the study of food as medicine, and lifestyle changes. The very things that helped me to overcome my own Epilepsy. My dad was the one who emphasized the importance of fitness and food as medicine when I was facing epilepsy as a 9-year-old. I began working out and eating good fats for my brain.

However, this book emphasizes ancient medicine and points out that our body is electric and that we have electrical circuits flowing through it, affecting our ability to stay healthy. If those circuits became blocked, it was just like a low battery affecting our health and performance. If this electricity was interrupted or blocked, then we could not reach our highest potential or have a high-performance body. I knew that day Ancient Medicine was the route I needed to take. Food as medicine, lifestyle changes, and the body's electricity were the answer. Even though Ancient Medicine had worked for 5,000 years, they did not teach any of this at UC Davis. So, I changed my major to Nutritional Science, graduated with a Bachelor of Science in NS, and then went on to Asian Medicine. I wanted to know more and help more people. To rebuild their bodies and brains and save their organs. I knew pharmaceuticals and surgery were not always the answer.

So, let me tell you a little about the body's electrical system. We have more nerves outside the body than inside. These are the electrical pathways from the skin to the internal organ systems. There are 14 major circuits from the top of your head to the bottom of your feet. I studied kinesiology, which is the study of muscles and circuits and how they relate to a healthy nervous system and a healthy body. It is this technique of diagnostics and testing that allows me to determine more specifically what is wrong with the body and what it needs nutritionally to be healthy and well. This knowledge is vital in very complex conditions.

The body needs two things: power and power flow. We get battery power from breathing, food, rest, water, nutrition, grounding, and positive thoughts. Grounding restores an electrical connection with the earth. I believe this connection has been lost in modern industrial society, in which people spend most of their time wearing shoes with rubber soles or living indoors. Earthing is a technique some people use to connect their physical bodies to the earth's electrical energy. Planet Earth has a negative electric charge. Some scientists theorize that free electrons are transferred to the human body during grounding.[74]

So, what negatively affects the electrical circuits in the body? Number one is scars; scars block the electrical flow of the body. Even a scar you got at 3 years old can block a circuit when you're 50.

---

[74] Bence, Sarah. "Grounding: Its Meaning, Benefits, and Exercises to Try." Edited by Melissa Bronstein. Verywell Health, June 14, 2023. https://www.verywellhealth.com/grounding-7494652.

One scar can affect many organs in the body. Another cause of an electrical problem would be dehydration and lack of electrolytes. When we don't get enough water, our organs don't function properly.

Another factor is minerals in the body, which are like spark plugs that keep the engine running. You can have the greatest engine in the world, but without spark plugs, it will never run, even if you have a full tank of gas.

The other factors that affect us electrically are toxins such as chemicals, metals, radiation, and even 5G. All of these affect our ability to function, and they must be removed to be able to restore function in our bodies.

Understanding The Electricity in your Body

Your body is like a battery; it needs electricity to keep your circuits running smoothly, and water is one of the best conductors. Remember that your body is more than 70% water and the brain more than 75% water. The human heart is electric. The human brain is electric, and every muscle in the human body is electric.

When someone has a neurological disease, it means there is a break somewhere in the body's electrical circuitry. The heart, brain, and/or muscles are no longer working in sync, which causes significant problems somewhere in the body.

Your body's electrical system has the potential to break down. Think about someone with a serious spinal injury. No matter what caused the injury, it resulted in an interruption or damage to the electrical system. Consider it this way – what would happen if you were struck several times by lightning? Now imagine those same lightning strikes inside your body, attacking your electrical wiring. Think of the damage it would do. It might seem improbable, but that is exactly what can happen. Let's put this in terms of electric potential. Think of a car battery – it has two terminals, one positive and one negative. When a car battery is fully charged, it can produce a higher voltage level than a small AA or AAA battery, for example.

Western medicine has a limited view of the electrical system, because it only tests 3 key areas of the body: the heart, the brain, the nerves, and the muscles. Asian medicine believes all of these, along with the cells, tissues, and organs, are an electrical network of batteries and circuits. Each organ is linked to certain meridians in the body. For example, the upper cartilage of the ear is linked to the uterus. Complications with this link prevented fertility in one of my patients. As soon as she took her earring out, she got pregnant. This is a key example of how important it is to know the electrical circuits of the body.

Scars and Electrical Flow

Scars on the body or within the body can block the healing process in many ways. Acupuncture is fantastic for resolving pain, yet it won't work for some people if there are active scars blocking the electrical flow in the body. I discovered this early in my practice. A man came to me for acupuncture to alleviate his pain, but he had over 50 surgeries throughout his life. He had so many scars, internally and externally, that acupuncture wouldn't help him until we worked on his scars.

When there are scars inside the body, it is parallel to a circuit being out on an electrical panel. It blocks the electrical flow, and the organs cannot function at full capacity. There are many kinds of scars. Some are tattoos or piercings. Others can be birthmarks or the result of injuries or surgeries of any kind. Internal scarring can be found with conditions such as endometriosis, car accidents, or physical trauma. Any scar that cuts across the meridians of the electrical pathways can potentially interfere with something inside the body. Asian medicine focuses on the electrical points in the body and how each point is connected to a function in the body. A panel of circuits that determine the electrical flow of each point and system in the body.

If you went to the electric panel to your house, opened it up, and discovered a circuit out, you would immediately know and understand that the panel outside affects the electricity inside. This is no different than our skin. Skin is the meeting point of the flow of electricity from the inside to the outside and the outside to the inside. This is known as the body's electrical field.

There are 5 Different Types of Flow in the Body:

- **Blood Flow,** which flows in a circle. Keeping the blood flowing and circulating is extremely vital to our health. A body in motion stays in motion.

- **Lymphatic Flow** is the body's detox mechanism. The Lymphatic system gets rid of toxins between cells, skin, and muscles. The toxins are released through exercise and muscle contractions. Getting a massage is a great way to release toxins from the lymphatic system. This flow is top to bottom, which means it's controlled and flows with gravity.

- **Mind Flow:** Your mind can control your body. If you think negative thoughts, then you become a negative person.

This will affect your physiology. It is what it is. If you're a positive person, you will affect your body in a positive way. Our thoughts affect our body, and our body affects our mind. This is the flow of the mind-body connection.

- **Glymphatic Flow:** The brain releases fluid to flush out the toxins and drain the glymphatic system. When you are asleep, the space between your brain cells increases, allowing fluid to flow freely. This is the brain-cleansing system. The glymphatic system opens during sleep, letting fluid flow rapidly through the brain. In a 2013 study, Dr. Maiken Nedergaard, M.D. and her team discovered that the glymphatic system helps control the flow of cerebrospinal fluid (CSF), a clear liquid surrounding the brain and spinal cord.[75] "We need sleep. It cleans up the brain," she said.

- **Electrical Flow:** This flow refers to the electrical flow through specific meridians, like blood vessels. This electrical flow is a pathway known and acknowledged by ancient medicine for thousands of years. Electrical flow is influenced by everything we do: our stress levels, how much we drink and exercise, how much food we eat before bed, and how much sleep we get. In Asian medicine, it is called the body's chi or vital energy. Our body is like one huge battery, and this is why grounding greatly helps our body. Our bodies are from the earth. You may or may not believe this, but science has conceded it is possible that our cells originated from a clay-like substance.

---

[75] "Brain May Flush out Toxins during Sleep." National Institutes of Health, September 17, 2015. https://www.nih.gov/news-events/news-releases/brain-may-flush-out-toxins-during-sleep.

"And the LORD God formed man from the dust of the ground,
and breathed into his nostrils the breath of life,
and man became a living soul."
–Genesis 2:7

That is why grounding is so beneficial. The earth has its own electrical flow, and so do we, and in this way, through grounding, we become one with the earth. (Earthing, also known as grounding, is when your bare skin – typically the feet – contacts the earth.)

- Each of our cells is like a battery within a bigger battery: our body, sitting on the world's largest battery, the earth. All of these batteries have electrical power and flow, so our bodies respond when grounding.

In 2017, atheists and scientist Richard Dawkins suggested human beings were born when mud in the form of clay learned how to replicate itself, ultimately leading to the creation of the famous DNA double helix and life itself.[76] Biological Engineers from Cornell University's Department for Nanoscale Science in New York State agreed clay 'might have been the birthplace of life on Earth'.[77]

Western Science

Many tools are used to measure electricity in the body, such as the EKG, the ECG, and so on. There's also a muscle nerve conduction test that is done, but it can be very painful. We know through science

---

[76] Baldwin, Paul. "REVEALED: How Life on Earth Began – and the Answer Is Even Crazier than You Thought." *Express UK*. August 17, 2017. https://www.express.co.uk/news/world/752936/Humans-evolved-from-MUD-says-Richard-Dawkins-bible-was-right-evolution-bible.

[77] Cornell University. "Clay may have been birthplace of life on Earth, new study suggests." ScienceDaily. www.sciencedaily.com/releases/2013/11/131105132027.htm (accessed July 19, 2024).

that all cells are electric. They communicate with each other, and it is critical to have good electrical flow between the cells, so that our body can operate at an optimum level without pain and with energy.

When our electrical system fails to function at this optimum level, sickness ensues, such as cancer, pneumonia, and COVID-19 etc. We must keep our electrical capability up and flowing properly. We are truly like a battery with circuits. We must keep the battery of the body charged on a cellular level. The battery of each cell is called the *mitochondria*. If the mitochondria are weak or disabled, we become weak and disabled. Many diseases and autoimmune conditions are caused by a depleted and failing mitochondria.[78] Each one of our cells creates an electric field outside of our body and together in unison. We have an electric, electromagnetic field around us. Often called the *morphogenic field* of the body. Think of it like a cat's whiskers or the ability to feel something late at night when walking down the hallway. It may be pitch black, but we can feel the wall even though we can't see it.

Kinesiology

The art of feeling the energy around the body or from within the body is a technique I often use in my clinic. This is a technique that goes back 100 years. This is the ability to use a muscle to measure electricity and electrical flow in the body and outside the body. We can find the acupuncture point like a circuit on the skin's surface with applied pressure. This technique is unfamiliar to many but backed by science and very effective.

---

[78] "What Are Mitochondrial Diseases?" Cleveland Clinic. Accessed July 19, 2024. https://my.clevelandclinic.org/health/diseases/15612-mitochondrial-diseases.

The Three Tests:

1. The heart is one of the most frequently tested parts of the body. Your doctor uses an Electrocardiogram (EKG or ECG) to measure the body's electrical flow. This records electrical signals from the heart and its rhythm, testing for many different heart conditions and telling doctors if the heart is damaged. If the EKG is abnormal, it tells you there is a problem with the heart's electrical connections.

2. The second most tested area is the brain, which is measured through an electroencephalogram (EEG). These tests measure electrical waves and activity in the brain and are used to determine conditions such as epilepsy, and that's how I found out that, as a child, I was epileptic. Later in life, the same tests told me that my brain activity was normal, and I no longer had epilepsy.

3. The third test and the most painful of all is the Electromyography (EMG). This test measures the electrical signals in your nerves and muscles, at rest and in use, to determine disorders such as muscular dystrophy, Guillain-Barre Syndrome, and carpal tunnel syndrome.

Biofeedback is a mind-body technique for controlling body functions, such as heart rate, breathing patterns, and muscle responses. During biofeedback, electrical pads are attached to the body to collect information about it.

The Electrical Potential

What creates electrical potential? That would be chemistry. It's all about how your cells are charged. Atomically speaking, the cells in our body control the electrical currents. Every element in the human body, such as potassium, calcium, sodium, and magnesium, has an electrical charge, and virtually every cell uses these charged elements, known as ions, to generate the electricity the body needs.

A membrane protects the cell's contents and is made of lipids that only allow certain substances to penetrate the interior. These lipids do two things – first, they stop certain molecules from getting in, and second, they help the cell generate those all-important electrical currents. How does this work? Well, resting cells have a negative charge on the inside, and their outside environment is positively charged. This is because the negative ions inside the cell and the positive ions outside are ever-so-slightly imbalanced. This charge separation is achieved by the cells allowing the ions to flow through the membrane in both directions. That flow generates our body's electrical currents, which can move at an impressive 120 meters per second.[79]

The cells in our bodies control how certain charged elements flow through the membrane by using proteins on the cell's surface to create openings for specific ions – these are called ion channels. Positive charges can get into the cell via these channels when each cell is stimulated. The interior of the cell is then positively charged, leading to more electrical currents, which, in turn, become electrical pulses known as action potentials. The human body uses specific action potential patterns to initiate the right behaviors, thoughts, and movements.

When those electrical currents are disrupted, things start to go wrong in the body. Let's take the heart as an example – for this to

---

[79] Raymond M Fish and Leslie A Geddes, "Conduction of Electrical Current to and through the Human Body: A Review," Eplasty, October 12, 2009, https://www.ncbi. nlm.nih.gov/pmc/articles/PMC2763825/.

pump properly, the cells need to generate the right current to ensure the heart contracts at the right time. That's where the EKG comes in, allowing doctors to see what's going on and prevent conditions like heart attacks.

What is Acupuncture?

Acupuncture is an ancient Chinese medical technique for relieving pain, addressing disease, and improving general health. It was devised before 2500 BCE in China and was used in many other areas of the world by the late 20th century. Acupuncture consists of inserting one or several small metal needles into the skin and underlying tissues at precise points on the body.

Structured Water and the "Exclusion Zone" (EZ)

Structured water ($H3O2$) can be considered a fourth state of water between liquid and solid. It has the hexagonal structure of ice; however, missing a critical bond, it behaves more like a gel than a solid, but retains some of its crystalline structure. Structured water can also drive fluid flow, so it may even be at least partly responsible for the flow in the meridians. $H3O2$ grows spontaneously next to hydrophilic (water-loving) surfaces. It grows layer upon layer, making what can be considered a very fine mesh that pushes out all impurities.

Inserting a Needle

A stainless-steel needle is hydrophilic by its very nature. So, when inserted in the body, it meets extracellular fluid, which is mostly water. An EZ then begins to form around the needle. This process is driven by radiant energy (mostly infrared energy or heat). Since the body has plenty of heat, this reaction occurs spontaneously. Because the concentration of protons grows in the surrounding water, it also becomes lower in pH. The negative charge of the EZ draws water molecules to it to continue the buildup of the EZ region, but also draws water to the site it's needed most.

What is Acupuncture Good For?

Acupuncture treatment, with its roots in traditional Chinese medicine, offers a versatile approach to health and well-being. Here are some acupuncture uses and benefits:

1. **Pain Management:**
    Acupuncture medicine has shown effectiveness in alleviating various types of pain, such as lower back pain, knee pain, and migraines. It's thought to stimulate the release of endorphins, the body's natural pain relievers.

2. **Stress Reduction:**
    Many people turn to acupuncture for its potential to reduce stress and promote relaxation. Acupuncture needles are believed to stimulate points that release tension and improve the body's stress response.

3. **Nausea and Vomiting:**
    Research suggests that acupuncture can help mitigate nausea and vomiting, especially in individuals undergoing chemotherapy or dealing with morning sickness during pregnancy.

4. **Anxiety and Depression:**
    Some studies indicate that acupuncture may have a positive impact on anxiety and depression symptoms, by influencing neurotransmitter levels.

5. **Insomnia:**
   Acupuncture might aid in improving sleep quality by addressing underlying factors contributing to insomnia.

The Electrical Heart

Let's talk about the heart for a moment. As we all know, it is a muscle that pumps blood through the body. Many studies have been done on this life-giving muscle. The heart wouldn't have enough power to pump blood through the body without its electrical system. Our cells generate electricity, so the blood flowing through our body is also charged by our electrical system. The heart has a sinus node that sends out electrical signals to the heart, and depending on your age, weight, health, and fitness level, these stimuli can produce 60 to 100 beats per minute. The electricity then moves through the electrical pathways running through the heart, helping it to contract and pump blood through the body's circulation system. That is what keeps us alive.

Heart as a Pump (Circulation)

The heart is a pump that circulates your blood through the body. But there are other ways in which the blood flows besides the heart itself. You must keep moving your blood through exercise, deep breathing, and muscle contraction to avoid blood stagnation. In Chinese medicine, blood stagnation leads to stroke, heart attack, a blood clot, or an aneurysm.

The human body relies on a second system to pump blood back to the heart. This system involves small valves throughout the veins and muscle contractions. This happens from your skeletal muscles when you walk and move. The valves close when blood starts to flow in one direction, so that blood in the veins can only flow in the direction back to the heart, which is up the legs. When you squeeze your leg muscles to walk, stand, kick, and move about, the muscles squeeze the veins and force the blood to get moving.

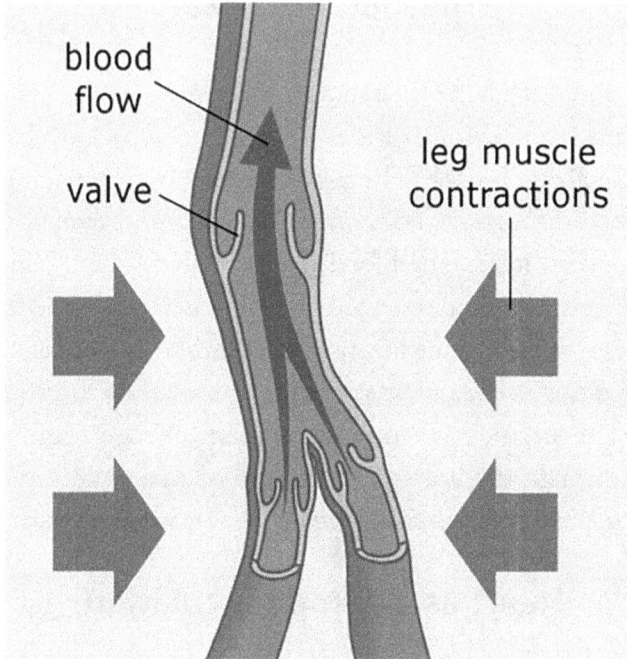

The heart is not strong enough by itself to get the blood back up the veins in your legs and back to your heart. The human body relies on a second system to finish that task. This system involves small valves throughout the veins and muscle contractions from your skeletal muscles when you walk and move about. The valves close when blood starts to flow in one direction so that blood in the veins can only flow in the direction back to the heart, which is up the legs.

When you squeeze your leg muscles to walk, stand, kick, and move about, the muscles squeeze the veins and force the blood to move. Because of the valves, the blood can only move in one direction as it gets squeezed along. So, it is a combination of blood pressure from the heart's pumping action, the valves, and muscle movement that gets the blood up the legs against gravity. If the valves malfunction, the blood begins to pool in the veins. This causes the veins to swell with blood, which can be painful and unsightly, known as varicose veins.

The harder the muscles work, the more vigorously the massive flow of blood generated by this activity returns to the heart.

This is why it is imperative to keep moving.

Fluid of the Heart-Blood: The Heart Chambers and Heart Valves

At the clinic, we have a specialized microphone called a Heart Sound Recorder that records and measures the sounds of the heart valves. I've learned that many of my patients have a problem with the efficiency of their heart valves. This problem does not always show up typically with an abnormal EKG but shows up ten to twenty years later as a leaky heart valve. The good news is if you take the right nutrition, such as whole foods supplements and vitamin B4, you can restore the function of the valve. Then, you will feel an increase in energy vitality, and your sleep will improve because your heart function will be more efficient.

Heart rate recovery (HRR) is how quickly your heart returns to normal after you stop exercising.[80] It is determined using your heart rate at the end of your workout and one minute later. This

---

[80] Braun, Ashley. "What Is Heart Rate Recovery?" Edited by Jeffrey S. Lander. Verywell Health, July 20, 2023. https://www.verywellhealth.com/heart-rate-recovery-5214767.

calculation is a measure of your physical fitness and an indication of your heart health.

The Brain Is Our Central Control System

Let's talk about the role the brain plays in the body. Everything we see, hear, smell, touch, and taste comes into our body, into this amazing electrical system we have, and the brain measures it to understand it; then, it can transfer what it learns to us. Every sense is related to a transformation that comes from chemical neurotransmitters created by neurons. The human body has many sensory, inter, and motor neurons. Individually, they are all constructed of different parts, but these neurons form a neural circuit when they are grouped together.

When these senses enter our body via our eyes, ears, mouth, nose, or body, they are transformed chemically and then sent to our brains. The final transformation occurs there, allowing us to understand that sense; it makes what we taste, hear, feel, and see real. In that sense, our body has one major language – electricity – and that is what talks to us. Think of this – when you close your eyes, sit at the edge of a pool, and dip your toes in. Your brain takes the sensation you feel, transforms it, and sends a signal back so that you understand what's happening. But the brain doesn't like using just one sense; it likes to use multiple senses simultaneously to ensure that you are not fooled by what you see, hear, taste, etc.

Another system like the EKG is the EEG, which measures brain waves. Like the heart, it's not possible to connect sensors directly to the brain, so sensors are placed on the scalp. Typical electrical signals in the brain are measured via the scalp at 30 to 50 microvolts. When they differ, the doctors can determine medical conditions like the epilepsy I was diagnosed with.

The Qi Phenomena

Let me tell you something. I've been practicing holistic healing for nearly 25 years, and 45 years ago, when I was just nine years old, I started studying nutrition. Over time, I learned that this electrical system in our bodies is called Qi (pronounced Chi). This name came from ancient practitioners after discovering the electrical connection, observing it, and learning about it.

In Eastern medicine, Qi is the vital energy that animates our bodies. When the electricity flows through the organs, it is named after them. So, for example, when it flows through the liver, it's called liver Qi, or kidney Qi when it flows through the kidneys. In Asian medicine, the differentiation is very important in terms of diagnosis. Like the electricity flowing through your house, we know that we can get electrical surges through our bodies. This overcharges the body and causes blockages in the circuitry; it's called Qi stagnation. Conversely, we could have too little electricity flowing through our bodies, which is known as Qi deficiency.

TCM Body Clock

TCM tells us that Qi is the most important thing. Qi commands our blood, and blood is the mother of Qi. That means blood is required to move Qi or energy around the body, but Qi already moves the blood. It's very much like the chicken and egg conundrum – which comes first – the blood or the Qi?

Back to the Beginning

When we are born, we are given the gift of life. But it goes back further than that, right to the point of conception. The egg and the sperm are both electrical. Multiple sperm try to reach the egg, but the first one there, the winner if you like, creates an electrical field that stops all the other sperm from penetrating the egg. Another electrical transformation occurs when that winning sperm penetrates the egg – the cells' electrical division.

Just stop and think for a moment – how much energy does it take to create a baby from one egg and one cell? How much energy does it take to grow that baby in the womb? Energy is akin to multiple lightning bolts, but we'll discuss that later.

Scars and Electrical Flow

The body is electric, and electrical issues in the body can be caused by several things, including scars – external scars, such as burns, moles, cuts, or surgical scars, and internal scars, like surgical scars or traumatic injuries from a car accident. These scars can block electrical flow in the body. I believe 5G, cell phones, cell phone towers, and other technologies can also cause electrical interference in the body. This is called electrical pollution; it's like a cloud of smog that damages our bodies.

First, I want to talk about scars and their effect on the electrical flow in the body. First, where does this electricity flow from? It comes from our cells, the body's energy and electricity powerhouse – we call it mitochondria. Those cells push that energy out to the rest of the body, creating body tissues and all those important organs we rely on for health and life – the heart, the lungs, the liver, the kidneys, and so on.

From there, that electricity flows to the meridian, the electrical circuit that runs right beneath the skin covering our bodies. Think of the meridian as a series of freeways or similar to the electrical wiring in your house. You can't see it, but you know it's there.

So, what happens if you cut yourself and your skin is scarred? Or if you get a tattoo, burn your skin, or undergo surgery? Every one of those scenarios can significantly affect that electrical circuit and how the electricity flows through your body. Look at it this way: if you cut through the electrical wires in your house, something will go wrong, and something will stop working. You could even create an electrical fire.

The same thing happens when your skin is scarred; you cut through or damage that all-important electrical circuit and something goes wrong. And yes, you could even create an electrical fire in your body, especially if the scarring is deep or bad. Most scarring heals eventually, but the electrical circuit damage still remains, which can bring problems. What if that circuit doesn't heal properly? If that happens, the electrical flow remains disrupted, often resulting in too much energy building up in the scar area.

If this happens, the energy can be discharged randomly, which can seriously upset your central nervous system, potentially resulting in serious issues that upset how your body works. What may seem to be a small scar can cause significant disruption if the energy builds up beneath it. In contrast, a large scar that you expect may not be a problem, especially if the electrical circuit heals as it should, and the energy doesn't build up.

Testimonial

I have been going to see Scott for five years. When I first met Scott, I had some very difficult digestive problems, and I was diagnosed with Crohn's Disease. I had allergy problems, both to food and to the environment. I have multiple bad discs in my back due to a work injury and have had serious pain. I also had heart issues, including a 60% blocked carotid artery. Scott evaluated me and began working on each problematic area.

Following Scott's treatments, I no longer have Crohn's disease. My ulcers have completely healed. He has treated my allergies using allergy clearing and supplements, which has helped tremendously. Scott has given me acupuncture treatments for my back and that has improved greatly as well. Finally, my carotid artery is no longer blocked, and I feel very strong. Before I went to see Scott, I was hardly able to leave the house and now I am feeling so much more able to have a full life. I didn't believe I would feel as well as I do now. Whether you come to Scott with health problems or are looking for a healthier lifestyle, Scott Sommer and his team are dedicated professionals. They gave me my life back. Thank you so much, Scott!

–Joe Antekeier

Tips:

- Get grounded to recharge your body's battery. To get grounded, go outside and touch the earth, ride horses, or walk barefoot on the grass. You can also touch the ground by your feet in a chair, lay on a blanket, or lean against a tree in a park.
- Get a grounding mat for your bed or desk.
- Drink lemon water with raw honey and a pinch of Redmond Real Salt®, or, if you prefer, drink coconut water

to help restore your electrolytes and balance your electrical flow.

- We continually use the Hugo therapy in the clinic to help restore electrical potential and the body's battery.
- We also carry a machine called BEMER therapy from Germany, which helps increase cellular energy and circulation.[81] It matches the electrical flow of the earth, so it's more powerful than a grounding mat.
- Start adding more organic minerals to your body by eating more organic fruits and vegetables and whole food supplements. Take trace minerals, vitamin B12, organically bound minerals, and Min Tran supplements (I suggest Standard Process Brand),
- Drink real water.
- Get some acupuncture from an experienced and highly trained TCM practitioner to help with electrical body balance, chronic pain, migraines, osteoarthritis, irritable bowel syndrome (IBS), and more.[82]
- Try the "Bed of Nails" acupressure massage technique. It reduces pain, minimizes stress, and improves circulation and sleep.[83]

The End

The end comes when the electricity flow stops. The energy stops when your life is over, and the spirit leaves your body. That spirit is

[81] Kreska, Zita et al. "Physical Vascular Therapy (BEMER) Affects Heart Rate Asymmetry in Patients With Coronary Heart Disease." *In vivo (Athens, Greece)* vol. 36,3 (2022): 1408-1415. doi:10.21873/invivo.12845.

[82] "Acupuncture: What You Need to Know." National Center for Complementary and Integrative Health. Accessed July 19, 2024. https://www.nccih.nih.gov/health/acupuncture-what-you-need-to-know.

[83] Day, Grace. "5 Benefits to Using Bed of Nails." Beauty Bay Edited, March 25, 2022. https://www.beautybay.com/edited/bed-of-nails-benefits/.

what creates that electrical flow together with your body. Together, they create that meridian, the electrical circuitry in your body, which gives you life. And it all starts at the point of conception, that breath of life that can be traced back to Adam and Eve, right back to when the Earth was created.

In that way, the breath of life is like a lightning bolt because it comes from above. It gives us life, which is the best gift anyone could ask for.

The more you read this book, the more you understand how your body works. When you understand that, you can understand your health and take control of it. Only you can ensure that your body stays healthy, and the electricity continues flowing smoothly through it.

Once you learn how the Qi works and how electricity helps you function, you will start feeling a sense of gratitude and wonder. It should even help you see how you can go on to help others in life, too.

I hope that understanding how electricity works will allow you to be grateful for how your body was created, how it works, and how it helps you function in life. It should even help you see how you can go on to help others in life, too.

One of the most awesome experiences you will ever have in life is having enough vitality and energy to do what you want to do, what you were created to achieve, and be in this life you were given. And this life? It's one to live to its fullest.

"We were created to heal and thrive.
Unfortunately, our society teaches that everything is fast food,
and fast medicine, which leads to fast disease.
It still takes sixty to ninety days to grow a tomato."
Scott Sommer, LAc

Scan the QR Code with your Smartphone to view message about: BODY IS ELECTRIC

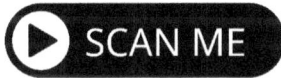

Or follow this link: https://qrco.de/ourelectricalbodies

Chapter 10

Energy

Let's talk about energy. We all know when we don't have much of it, but how many of us really know where it comes from? Of course, the obvious answer is the food we eat, but the reality is far more complex than that. So, how do we help ourselves power up when we are feeling down?

Get Outdoors

Our bodies get energy from multiple sources, the first being the sun. Most of us think that only plants need the sun to survive and give them the energy to grow, but we humans need it, too. The sun provides the body with something it cannot take on its own: vitamin D. Have you ever wondered why you feel so much more energetic and alive when you are out in the sun? When you don't have enough vitamin D in your body, your energy levels fall, and you feel like crap. Stand in the sun for a few minutes, and you feel those energy levels rising.

Breathe Deep

Breathing pulls oxygen into the body, providing us with energy. This is why many doctors and therapists recommend deep breathing as an exercise. Think of someone who isn't getting enough oxygen into their body, somebody choking, for example. Fast, shallow breathing or choking uses up the body's oxygen supplies very quickly, and if they cannot get enough back into the body, they could lose their life.

Drink That Water

Back in Chapter 2, we learned that sufficient hydration is critical for the human body's survival. Drinking enough water helps detox your body – you could see it as taking out the trash. It also helps rejuvenate the body's cells and transport nutrients where they need to go. Think about a time when you've felt tired and drained during the day. Is it because you didn't sleep well the night before? Is it because you haven't given yourself a break? Or is it because you simply didn't drink enough water? It's not just your body that needs water – your brain does, too, and your energy levels will plummet without that supply of hydration.

Eat the Right Food

This is the most common energy source, but it's not just about eating for fuel – it's about what you eat and when you eat it. The old saying, "You are what you eat," is incredibly true in this case. You can only get as much energy as the food you eat provides, and while you might think that a candy bar or fast-food burger is enough, it isn't. All food like that raises your blood sugar levels, boosting energy. But that burst doesn't last long because it falls very quickly when your blood sugar spikes. It's a vicious cycle – when your energy levels drop, you reach for another cookie or candy bar, so the cycle continues.

In Chapter 3, we learned how our food has changed drastically over the last century. Much of it is now modified in some way – it is full of salt, added sugar, preservatives, and so on – none of which is healthy.

Transforming the Body

One of the most important natural nutrients is iodine, which helps the thyroid and the metabolism function properly.[84] The thyroid is one of the human body's energy glands, the second being the adrenal gland. Together, they provide a source of transformation in the body, and that's what energy sources are all about – transformation.

Water is transformed into power – we know it as hydroelectricity in terms of external energy, but the same thing happens in the body. Water fuels our internal battery and helps electricity flow through our bodies.

Food is transformed in the body, too. Everything we eat breaks down into something the body can use and digest easily. The proteins you consume are broken down into amino acids, which are then converted into energy to fuel you. Those proteins help keep your nails, hair, eyes, and skin healthy too.

The fat you eat is broken down into tiny chains of fatty acids, which the body uses in many ways. First, it feeds the phospholipids that provide a membrane in the body's cells – these membranes regulate what can and cannot pass in and out of the cells. Weak membranes lead to being out of shape and lower energy levels. Fat also provides the body with protection in the form of warmth and stored calories. It gives us the energy we need, not just for the body but for the brain, too.

Most of you have heard of the keto diet and ketosis, but do you understand it? When the body is in ketosis, it burns fat rather than

---

[84] "Office of Dietary Supplements – Iodine." NIH Office of Dietary Supplements. Accessed July 19, 2024. https://ods.od.nih.gov/factsheets/Iodine-Consumer/.

glucose as fuel. The only way to get into ketosis is to drastically cut your carbohydrate intake and up your intake of protein and healthy fats. Protein and fat are transformed into useful things that your body needs: amino acids. There are at least eight types of amino acids.

Why We Need Energy

The simple answer to that is that we need the energy to function. The body uses it to function in everything we do. Every cell in the human body contains its powerhouse, called mitochondria, which helps produce energy. That energy powers the functions in our body, including:

- Waking up in the morning
- Digesting the food you eat
- Keeping your body warm and your heart beating
- Keeping you moving throughout the day, and
- Repairing skin cells

It also helps your cells reproduce as the old ones break down. Your red blood cells break down every 3 to 4 months, and if they aren't replaced with new ones, you will become anemic. The same occurs if they don't reproduce after an injury or damage.

Maintaining and Regulating Energy

Let's describe this in terms of a water tank. Water is best stored at an elevated position. The higher, the better. That way, there is enough pressure to distribute the goods to the town below. The more pressure there is, the more potential there is. This is the same as the electricity in our bodies. The cells in the body have a level of energy equivalent to 5 thunderbolts – that's a huge amount. If our cells didn't contain that energy, we would always be tired, lethargic, and unable to accomplish anything.

So, how does this energy flow through the body?

When someone has a blockage in their energy flow, it's known as Qi stagnation in Eastern medicine. This causes many problems in the body, and the only way to avoid it is to keep the energy flowing. That starts with the mind. We need to think positively and clearly. If our energy flow slows down or becomes blocked, it can cause swelling, pain, and discomfort. This leads to weight gain, where the abdominal fat becomes blocked. Exercise is another great way to regulate energy and stop the blockages.

Let's use another analogy – your body is a car that has run out of gas and is stranded by the roadside. The breakdown leaves you stuck – your car has no fuel to get going again, and you can't get to the store to buy the fuel your body needs to get going again.

You can't do anything if your body doesn't have a supply of energy. The human body is full of cells, trillions upon trillions of them, and every single one needs energy to fuel its mitochondria. That energy comes from food, water, and the air you breathe. It also comes from exercise, nutrients, and minerals.

Food is Energy

The human body is a powerhouse; it's as simple as that. When you let that powerhouse run out of fuel, it leads to exhaustion and illness. Sure, you can recharge it, but that takes a lot of time and isn't easy. This is why it is so important to keep the energy flowing through your body so that it gets distributed to the right places.

Each cell is a tiny battery in that powerhouse, and they are all connected somehow. Together, they produce the incredible amount of energy we use. These cells are a big part of the human body's nervous system, constantly running in the background without us even thinking about it. They control our temperature, blood pressure, and how the heart pumps the blood around our body, all the things we take for granted.

In Asian medicine, our energy flow needs to find somewhere to go. So, each little battery or cell is connected through a circuit. These cells comprise our body tissues, which, in turn, make up our organs. The organs and glands use these circuits to communicate with one another, and these circuits are often called nerve pathways.

These pathways can be seen on an MRI scan. Just recently, a technological breakthrough was made when an acupuncture point was discovered using MRI.[85] This confirmed that these acupuncture points exist and are not the same as the other tissues in our bodies.

The electrical circuits that connect those cells are like freeways, full of energy whizzing about – the energy produced from the food we eat, the air we breathe, and the water we drink. Feeding your body with good, nutritious food and water creates energy that flows through your body, like water flowing to a farmer's crops.

I like to consider the electrical flow through our bodies, like water through the nerve pathways, like how blood flows through our veins, arteries, and capillaries.

---

[85] Parrish, Todd B et al. "Functional magnetic resonance imaging of real and sham acupuncture. Noninvasively measuring cortical activation from acupuncture." *IEEE engineering in medicine and biology magazine – the quarterly magazine of the Engineering in Medicine & Biology Society* vol. 24,2 (2005): 35-40. doi:10.1109/memb.2005.1411346.

Sadly, while energy is a critical factor in our lives, to our survival and wellbeing, most of us don't give it a second thought until our energy levels run low and our motivation disappears. A lack of energy can affect us in many ways – physically, mentally, emotionally, and even spiritually. We need the strength to keep pushing forward and deal with everything that heads our way.

Think about blood pumping through your body. It oxygenates the heart, flows through large vessels and into the smaller ones, and from there, it goes to all the capillaries in your body. But have you ever thought about what makes it flow? Where does the energy come from to propel it through your body?

Remember that model of the heart as a pump that we talked about? It showed that the heart didn't have sufficient energy to pump blood through the body. This means the body has another energy force that helps the heart push that blood around, keeping you alive: electricity, or Qi, the human body's life force.

Energy is created from birth. In TCM, we are born with a certain amount of energy called Jing, which is known as our genetic energy. The additional energy we acquire throughout life is like charging a battery each day. Here are some ways to increase your energy.

Tips

1. **Get restorative sleep.** As you sleep, your body repairs itself. You should wake up every morning rested, refreshed, and ready for the day. Great sleep equals great energy. (In chapter 11, I detail the value of sleep for overall health. Follow my sleep recommendations at the end of the chapter to further improve your energy levels throughout the day.)

2. **Hydration.** Drink pure water first thing in the morning. Below is a hydration recipe I call "The Shovel."

"The Shovel:"

- Pinch of Redmond Real Salt®
- .5-1 tsp. raw local honey
- .5- 1 tsp. extra virgin olive oil
- 1-3 tsp. apple cider vinegar
- Juice from half a lemon

Add all ingredients to 6-12 oz of warm water in the morning. Or drink warm lemon water with raw honey and a pinch of Redmond Real Salt®.

3. **Keep moving daily.** I have a saying; "keep moving to keep moving." Think of this: some species of sharks, like the great white, must keep moving, or they will die. We are like a great white shark. We must keep swimming. A sedentary life is unhealthy. If we don't stay active, we lose energy and become exhausted. If you don't keep moving and building muscle, you'll be unable to accomplish your goals. I suggest pushing yourself out of your comfort zone by exercising to build your stamina. I recommend HIT training or interval training.

4. **Remember to get enough rest and relaxation in your day.** Take 10-to-60 minute breaks throughout your day, and treat them like mini-vacations.

5. **Get energy from whole food.** One could say that we should eat more like a rabbit than a lion. This means that we always need to consume twice the number of vegetables to fruits, more quality

protein and less poor-quality meat (such as pork, Tilapia, and farm raised fish). Also, eat less grains and simple carbs. Avoid highly processed salt which may not have the right amount of minerals to keep your body healthy. Redmond Real Salt® helps your adrenal glands function better.

6. **Get at least 30-60 minutes of sunshine each morning.** Just take a moment to sit outside and relax in the sun. It it's too cold, sit near a window.

Testimonial

I have received acupuncture, foot detox baths, and great care with supplement support. Scott created an individualized plan for me based on my body's need for supplementation. I like this because no two people are alike so the program shouldn't be the same for each person. I like the atmosphere of the office; it is very peaceful. Looking forward to trying out some of the other treatments they offer in their office. Thanks, Sommer's Holistic Center for supporting my healthy journey!

A Miracle

The human body really is a miracle, full of systems, pathways, and electrical circuits that keep us alive and thriving. When even one of those circuits breaks down, it disrupts the rest of them, leading to disease.

The most important thing to remember is that energy is the core of life. We are given a gift when we are born: the breath of life. That gift is what propels us forward, kickstarting the whole growth process right from the moment of conception. The transformation starts when the egg meets the sperm, creating an incredible process robust enough to transform that egg and sperm into a fetus for a human being to be created and born into the world. The womb is a battery, surrounded and fed by electrical energy, providing the energy we need to survive.

The exact process works in the body, with our cells continually repairing and regrowing, reproducing billions daily.

Energy is vital to us. Energy equals life, and life equals energy. It is responsible for our longevity and vitality. Everything depends on how we restore our energy and ensure it is distributed around the body daily. It all depends on the food we eat, the exercise we choose, and how much rest we get. It depends on the nutrients and the water we take in.

Everything we take in and everything we do is critical. Think of it as riding an electric bike with electric wheels. The spokes are the electrical connections connecting to the rest of the body and our organs. We start pedaling that bike the moment we are conceived and continue pedaling it throughout our lives. Some people struggle to continue pedaling because they haven't paid attention to their health. Eating the right foods, exercising regularly, and living a healthy lifestyle will help you regain your energy.

And that is the whole point: If you don't take care of yourself, your life force, that energy or Qi, will falter and become blocked if you don't look after your body. If we don't keep pedaling, the energy will stop. Everything you do in life matters – what you eat, drink, do, how you live your life, even what and how you think. It all affects how you manage your energy to ensure you live a productive life.

Scan the QR Code with your Smartphone to view message about: Energy

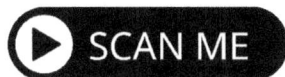

Or follow this link: https://qrco.de/body_energy

Chapter 11

Sleep

- Do you fall asleep in 5 or 10 minutes?
- Do you stay asleep?
- Do you wake up through the night?
- Do you wake up rested in the morning?
- Do you sleep with a CPAP machine?
- Do you fall asleep throughout the day? (Narcolepsy)
- Do you have difficulty falling asleep?

Most of us are unaware of how well we sleep unless we wake up during the night, can't fall asleep, or wake up tired. Statistically, we spend one-third of our lives sleeping, a tremendous amount of time in comparison to the time that we are awake. Studies show that sleep is directly related to the health of your heart. Longevity is based on how much we allow our bodies to sleep. Insomnia is linked to high blood pressure and heart disease.[86] Over time, poor sleep can hurt your heart, including higher stress levels, less motivation to be physically active, and unhealthy food choices.

Sleep equals repair and detox.

---

[86] "About Sleep and Your Heart Health." Centers for Disease Control and Prevention. Accessed July 19, 2024. https://www.cdc.gov/heart-disease/about/sleep-and-heart-health.html?CDC_AAref_Val=https%3A%2F%2Fwww.cdc.gov%2Fbloodpressure%2Fsleep.htm.

Amazing Breakthrough!

Scientists have discovered a revolutionary new treatment that makes you live longer. It enhances your memory and makes you more creative. It makes you look more attractive. It keeps you slim and lowers food cravings. It protects you from cancer and dementia. It wards off colds and the flu. It lowers your risk of heart attacks and stroke, not to mention diabetes. You'll even feel happier, less depressed, and less anxious. Are you interested? The evidence supporting these claims has been documented in more than 17,000 well-scrutinized scientific reports to date. As for the prescription cost, well, there isn't one. It's free. Yet all too often, we shun the nightly invitation to receive our full dose of this all-natural remedy – with terrible consequences.

The second benefit of sleep for memory comes after learning, one that effectively clicks the "save" button on those newly created files. In doing so, sleep protects newly acquired information, affording immunity against forgetting: an operation called consolidation.
–Matthew Walker PhD, Why We Sleep

Quotes by Matthew Walker

"Sleep is the Swiss army knife of health. When sleep is deficient, there is sickness and disease. And when sleep is abundant, there is vitality and health.

"Human beings are the only species that deliberately deprive themselves of sleep for no apparent gain. Many people walk through their lives in an under-slept state, not realizing it."

"Regularity is a key: going to bed at the same time, waking up at the same time no matter what. But I think, also, it's not just about quantity – that's what we've been discovering. It's also about quality."

"Alcohol is a class of drugs that we call 'the sedatives.' And what you're doing is just knocking your brain out. You're not putting it into natural sleep."

"Sleep is Mother Nature's best effort yet to counter death."

Back in the 1940s, people were sleeping on average just a little bit over eight hours a night, and now, in the modern age, we're down to around 6.7, 6.8 hours a night.

During sleep, many processes in the body are active that are inactive during the day, like an instrument in an orchestra repairing the hormones and organs.

Cortisol: It increases as we sleep, specifically so we can wake up alert. Cortisol acts as a stimulant during the day, then drops off at night to allow us to sleep.

Cortisol's Natural Rhythm: Our bodies follow a natural circadian rhythm for cortisol, with levels peaking in the early morning (around 3 am) to promote alertness upon waking. As the day unfolds, cortisol levels gradually diminish, reaching their low point at night. *(https://www.ptsduk.org/sleep-and-cortisol-)*

Melatonin is the only known hormone synthesized by the pineal gland and is released in response to darkness, hence the name "hormone of darkness." When you turn off the lights, melatonin is released int the body to help you fall asleep. However, many people struggle to create this environment as many things today interfere with this natural process, such as blue light, TV, video games, and noise, both inside and out. Melatonin provides a circadian and seasonal signal to the organisms in vertebrates.[87]

---

[87] Masters, Alina et al. "Melatonin, the Hormone of Darkness: From Sleep Promotion to Ebola Treatment." *Brain disorders & therapy* vol. 4,1 (2014): 1000151.

Many have found white noise helpful in drowning out the snoring of a spouse, sirens, barking dogs, etc. It is best to avoid your cell phones, TVs, and computers right before bed. You must create the right environment to fall asleep. If you fail to sleep enough, your body will break down and age. Very fast. One of the ways this shows up in our clinic is by measuring the HRV of the body. The biological age of your body.

The HRV (Heart Rate Variability) measures your heart rhythm and compares it to over half a million people, from Olympic athletes to people on their deathbeds. This is a type of biofeedback like a blood pressure cuff measuring your blood pressure. Two numbers are assessed from the test, including your estimated Physiological age and how fast your body is aging compared to your biological age. Sometimes, patients are discouraged by their body age, yet it's important to know if you are getting close to the edge of disease so you can self-correct. You can change the direction of your health when you are faced with the truth.

Success Story

"I'm truly grateful I found Dr. Sommer and received treatment at the healing center. I wasn't sleeping more than 2 to 3 hours a night, and it was really taking a toll on my health!

My GP doctor said it was stress and anxiety and prescribed medication. I just wasn't feeling any better, so a friend recommended Dr. Sommer's Holistic Healing. After a few weeks of treatments and supplements, I felt so much better!! Back to sleeping 6 to 8 hours a night. My hormones are much better now, and I'm thinking more clearly!

---

doi:10.4172/2168-975X.1000151.

Dr. Scott is the real deal, and their staff is caring and very efficient! We have more work to do, but I'm thankful to have my health back on a great path!! I hope this will help someone who needs it!
–Kim Gordon

My goal is to inspire you to self-correct and know that your DNA is not your destiny.

I ask new patients, "How do you sleep?" Their response? "Not great. I wake up 3 to 5 times a night." Sleep is like a symphony of signals that must be in complete harmony. In Asian medicine, we look at the circadian clock. Circadian rhythms are the physical, mental, and behavioral changes an organism experiences over a 24-hour cycle. Light and dark influence circadian rhythms, but food intake, stress, physical activity, social environment, and temperature also affect them.[88]

In Asian and Western medicine, the liver plays a big role in our ability to sleep, repair, and detox. I use the analogy of a repairman (your liver) showing up in the middle of the night to repair all the damage that occurred during the day. Then, when you wake up in the morning, you're fully rested and restored, ready for action the next day. It is like recharging your battery and ensuring the engine is ready for the next drive.

Each day should be like an Easter egg hunt. We should intentionally collect nutrition throughout the day, which can be used for repair, detox, and restoration at night during the sleep cycle.

---

[88] "Circadian Rhythms." National Institute of General Medical Sciences. Accessed July 19, 2024. https://www.nigms.nih.gov/education/fact-sheets/Pages/circadian-rhythms.aspx.

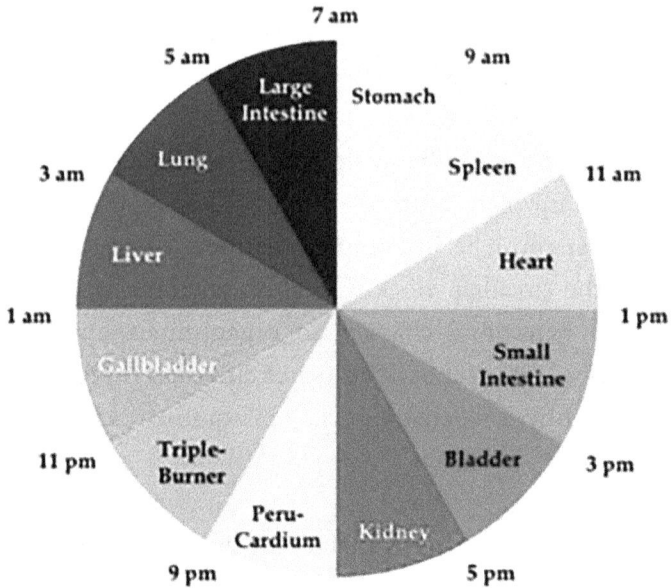

Chinese Model

The clock is based on a 24-hour time period, and each organ corresponds to a two-hour interval when it's most abundant and strong. As mentioned, the time *opposite* each organ's interval is when it is at its weakest energetic point. This relative strength and weakness is reflective of one of the main underlying principles in TCM: balance.

The most significant aspect of the body clock is its ability to explain how it functions at certain times of day to maintain wellness and fight disease. The TCM body clock tells us when it is best to eat, sleep, and exercise, among many other things.

Below, you will find a simple chart that states the two-hour interval, the organ with its highest functioning state, and a box for considering the organ's clock opposite the time when it is weakest.

You will also read some comments about emotions. Specific emotions are inherently connected with organs in TCM, which also link to times of the day. For example, many people tend to wake up between 3-5 am, during the Lung time. The emotion associated with the Lungs is grief or worry, so we hear a lot of patients say they wake up during that time of the night worrying or feeling sad.

The first twelve hours involve TCM organs that have actions that help us have a healthy and productive day. (For example, respiration, elimination, taking in, digesting, and assimilating nutrients, building blood, strong mental-emotional health, etc.) As the day starts to wind down and our activity (should) become less, the next twelve-hour period sees qi move through organs that have a lot of functions in storing, protecting, repairing, and balancing the body.

Everything we do during the day affects our sleep during the night.

If we eat light and intentionally do those things that will improve our sleep, we will begin to see changes in our sleep. *Sleep equals rest, detox, and repair.* Blood sugar also affects sleep, so eating desserts and drinking wine before bed can work against you. You may fall asleep, but high blood sugar can cause you to wake up two hours later.

Those with either sleep apnea or disrupted sleep patterns had higher blood glucose levels. People with the most severe sleep apnea had 14% higher blood glucose levels than those without it.[89] Sleep issues are one of the most complex issues in the body. Sleep involves shifts in hormones and minerals, and minerals such as calcium and magnesium play a crucial role.

"A lack of the nutrients calcium and magnesium will cause you to wake up after a few hours and not be able to return to sleep."[90]

Blood sugar also plays a big role in how well we sleep. The liver and the pancreas play a tennis match during the night. Blood sugar interferes with sleep. Sleep problems are one of the deepest issues of the body because sleep causes so many different hormonal shifts and minerals. There are necessary pathways that must be open to get quality sleep. Minerals such as calcium and magnesium also play a big role.

You can order fantastic pure minerals from us or purchase top-notch quality minerals from another source. Be on a nutritional easter egg hunt to gather nutrition throughout the day to use at night for proper detox, restoration, and sleep. The proper sleep environment is vital, so make sure you have a window cracked for fresh air or get a home-filtering air purifier. Make sure to keep the room cold, dark, quiet, and peaceful.

[89] *News in Health*, July 2020. https://newsinhealth.nih.gov/2020/07/poor-sleep-linked-higher-blood-sugar.

[90] "Medical and Health Information | Medicalnewstoday." Medical News Today. Accessed July 19, 2024. https://www.medicalnewstoday.com/releases/163169#1.

Success Story

Before seeing Scott, I had issues with sleeping & had to take Benadryl every night for 4 years just to go to sleep. Scott helped me to get off the Benadryl & now my body has been regulated and I am able to fall asleep without taking any toxic substances.
–Corrie Enriquez

Creating the Right Sleep Environment is Very Important

8 Tips to Improve Sleep:

1. Start exercising. If you can't walk, then do chair exercises. Walking, stretching, cycling, and running will all improve your sleep.
2. Avoid caffeine later in the day.
3. Darken your room- Melatonin is released.
4. Crack a window for fresh air.
5. Don't use electronic devices before bed.
6. Try using white noise, such as a fan or white noise device.
7. Take Calcium or Magnesium before bed.
8. Enjoy a protein snack before bed instead of a sugary one. I sleep great when I wake up between 3:00 and 5:00 a.m., grab something to eat, and go to the bathroom.

Now that you have some great tips on improving your sleep, you can start enjoying a more restful sleep and wake up refreshed and full of energy.

Scan the QR Code with your Smartphone
to view message about: Sleep

Or follow this link: https://qrco.de/ImportanceofSleep

Chapter 12

Bones, Muscles, and Movement

Bones and muscles in the body are like the body and tires on a car. Without them, you can't get from one place to another. You must understand the fundamentals of the body's functions to recognize when it fails to function. Strong muscles and bones enable you to live a vibrant life. Weak muscles and bones rob you of your independence and limit what you can do. Your muscles get weaker gradually over time as you age. First, you need help opening a jar, and then, over time, you have difficulty walking and lifting things. When walking becomes difficult, many are forced to use a cane or a walker. Much of the population falls after age 60 simply because their legs are too weak to sustain them. Falls and breaks can be devastating to our lives as we age.

My Aunt

I remember my aunt Emma, a good, strong German woman who was self-sufficient her entire life. One day, we got the call that she had lost her balance, fell, and shattered her hip. She lost her independence and had to live in an assisted care home from then on, and her life was forever changed.

She fell because her legs were weak, and she had no muscle strength to sustain her. Aunt Emma had a typical American diet full of acidic foods that pulled calcium out of her bones. Aunt Emma could no longer be active or do the things she loved, like gardening. She spent the rest of her days immobile, tired, and depressed. This is a common scenario. Over time, she lost the muscle in her legs, affecting her balance. To make matters worse, she didn't do any weight-bearing exercises to build bone density. Gradually, over a 10 to 20 year period, she developed osteoporosis.

Unfortunately, like my aunt, many of us are unaware of this decline happening under our skin. Many diseases like this develop over extended periods of time.

How Muscles Work

There are about 600 muscles in the human body.[91] Muscles have a range of functions, from pumping blood and supporting movement to lifting heavy weights or giving birth. Muscles work by either contracting or relaxing to cause movement. Muscles equal metabolism, movement, and energy production. As your muscles grow stronger from exercise, they pull harder on bones. The harder they tug, the more your body strengthens those bones. The reverse is also true.

If you don't work out, your muscles get weaker each decade, and the force they apply to your bones diminishes. Building your muscles daily is like making daily deposits into your bones and future mobility. In summary, the more you exercise your muscles, the stronger your bones will be.

The aging process is inevitably accompanied by structural and functional changes in vital organs. Skeletal muscle, which accounts for 40% of total body weight, plays crucial physical and metabolic roles

---

91 Department of Health & Human Services. "Muscles." Better Health Channel, March 12, 2010. https://www.betterhealth.vic.gov.au/health/conditionsandtreatments/muscles.

in humans.[92] Sarcopenia is a condition characterized by significant loss of muscle mass and strength. It is related to subsequent frailty and instability in the elderly population.[93] As we get older, our bones typically get more fragile as well. You must keep moving to keep moving.

Bones and muscles are directly connected to movement, which determines your ability or inability to enjoy your life. Understanding the importance of this will hopefully motivate you to start moving, strengthening, and building each of these. That is my goal to inspire and motivate you. It's never too late unless it's too late. Every skyscraper needs a firm foundation. Most skyscrapers are built deep into the earth with pylons to keep them from toppling over. Our bodies are no different. Like a skyscraper, our body needs a firm foundation from the legs up. Our bones are living tissue, and they can grow and replace old bones in about 10 years.[94] Without our bones, there would be nothing to protect our brains or organs.

Think about your feet. Your feet are the foundation for your entire body. They allow your body to balance, stand, walk, run, and jump and absorb damaging shock that enters your body every time your heel hits the ground.[95] That means if you have problems with

---

[92] Frontera, Walter R, and Julien Ochala. "Skeletal muscle: a brief review of structure and function." *Calcified tissue international* vol. 96,3 (2015): 183-95. doi:10.1007/s00223-014-9915.

[93] Ardeljan, Andrew D., and Razvan Hurezeanu. "Sarcopenia." National Library of Medicine, January 2024. https://www.ncbi.nlm.nih.gov/books/NBK560813/#:~:text=Sarcopenia%20is%20a%20musculoskeletal%20disease,system%20or%20impair%20physical%20activity.

[94] Office of the Attorney General, Bone Health and osteoporosis: A report of the Surgeon General. executive summary § (2004). https://www.ncbi.nlm.nih.gov/books/NBK45513/.

[95] Milcarek, Erica. "Your Feet Are Your Foundation." Active Spine & Joint, March 21, 2022. https://www.activespineandjoint.com/activesj-blog/your-feet-are-your-foundation.

your feet, your entire body will suffer. You can experience knee, hip, and lower back pain with ongoing foot problems. Foot issues can also cause imbalance, poor posture, and more.[96] Good foot health is essential for an active life.

"Keep striving for better yet! Never settling, always reaching for better yet."
–Scott Sommer, LAc

Story
Jumping is Fun

One Saturday afternoon, my two daughters (who were very young at the time) and I were on the trampoline in our backyard. They challenged me to jump rope on the trampoline. I said, "You're on!!!" We practiced and counted who of us could jump the longest. This tradition has become a part of my daily exercise routine to this day, under our redwood trees while watching the sunrise. I believe this should be a part of the Olympics. I believe this is the best aerobic and anaerobic exercise I have ever done in my life so far. I can do 5-10 minutes on the trampoline jump rope and feel like I went to the gym for an hour. Please do not try this unless you feel you are physically able to do this combo exercise (you must have good balance and a strong heart).

You can bounce your way into better balance, bones, muscles, and circulation.[97] Start jumping on an outdoor or mini trampoline daily (hold on to the bar if needed). If you have small children, we recommend a guard railing around the outdoor trampoline and a

---

[96] "Plantar Fasciitis & Foot Pain." Active Spine & Joint. Accessed July 19, 2024. https://www.activespineandjoint.com/conditions/plantar-fasciitis-foot-pain.

[97] Cleveland Clinic. "Health Benefits of Exercising on a Trampoline." Cleveland Clinic, July 2, 2024. https://health.clevelandclinic.org/trampoline-workout-benefits.

bar on the mini trampoline. Rebounding is a full-body workout that impacts your whole body. Plus, all the jumping will make you feel like a kid again.

Benefits of Trampoline Exercise:

- Builds strength by engaging all of your muscles simultaneously-including your abs, legs, back, and a strong core and beyond.
- Improves bone density. Our bones become more fragile with age unless we stress them with exercise.

Bones, muscles, and movement allow us to have mobility in our joints. They all work together to ensure a smooth flow. Muscles are connected and attached to bones via tendons to strengthen the bones through tension. Together, they work much like a guitar. Muscles like the strings of the guitar create flexibility and tension, and movement to create sound, yet they must have the structure of the guitar, like bones in the body, to create music.

So strong muscles make strong bones work together in harmony (get it?), to create a high-performance body. One without the other would be without purpose. It truly amazes me how we were so thoughtfully made... have you ever thought about being grateful to have muscle and bones working together for your best self. All you have to do is feed them and work to keep them working efficiently and effectively for a vibrant life with a divine purpose and plan.

Research shows that muscles are connected to the mitochondria (the battery inside each cell). The mitochondria live inside the cells of your muscles and create energy. When you exercise, the body responds by making more mitochondria to keep up with the energy requirement. It also stimulates autophagy, which helps to rid the body of damaged cells. In short, exercise helps increase and optimize the function of the mitochondria.

When the mitochondria is damaged or breaking down, autoimmune conditions often develop. So, exercising is necessary not only for a high-performance body but also for maintaining the health of your cells. In my clinical experience, I've heard repeatedly that most people don't exercise. Many people feel too tired or unwell to exercise regularly. Some think others only exercise to better their appearance, and just decide there's no point in trying.

Yet, soon, the consequences catch up with them in the form of disease. Our bodies were designed to move and to keep moving. Movement keeps your blood flowing and increases the oxygen in your blood. You must find the time to exercise to avoid the consequences. Stagnant blood is like a polluted swamp where disease just grows and festers. Stagnant blood lacks oxygen, and a lack of oxygen in the blood can lead to cancer. According to a 2012 University of Georgia study, low oxygen levels in cells may be a primary cause of uncontrollable tumor growth in some cancers.[98]

Cancer has difficulty surviving in an oxygen-rich environment if the blood moves like a river or bubbling spring. So exercise not only enables you to live and move, but it also prevents disease. Aging leads to bone loss, so you must focus on weight-bearing exercises to prevent bone loss and increase bone density. Every part of our body is interconnected and dependent upon each other.

---

[98] University of Georgia. "Low oxygen levels could drive cancer growth, research suggests." ScienceDaily. www.sciencedaily.com/releases/2012/05/120503194219. htm (accessed July 19, 2024).

Muscles and Energy

Building muscle boosts energy because it increases the mitochondria (battery of the cell) in the muscle cells, resulting in strength and power in your overall physique. The more muscle you have, the more energy you'll have, and the less caffeine you will need. When you get the blood flowing, it produces oxygen in the blood, which in turn produces energy. People who exercise regularly have more energy than people who don't. Consistent exercise and eating right can help manage common conditions like chronic fatigue. Keep that in mind before running to the next pharmaceutical with negative side effects.

If you suffer from fatigue and this feels overwhelming to you, just start walking. Start with 5 minutes a day and try to increase your time day by day. Baby steps are the key to change; remember this quote: *"Inch by inch change is a cinch, yard by yard change is hard."*

The positive side effects of exercise are feeling fantastic, strong, and living life to its fullest. Think about that. This should inspire you to start exercising daily as soon as you can. Sarcopenia is the loss of muscle mass that occurs after the age of 30 and continues as we age. Muscles decrease by 3 to 8% every decade, reaching 50% by age 80.[99] Many bone conditions also develop, such as osteoporosis and osteopenia, so building muscle as we age is very important. This decline of muscle occurs rapidly unless we play an active role in preventing it, so if you want to be mobile, you must work fervently to keep your muscles. Weight-bearing exercises increase muscle and prevent bone loss.

---

[99] Volpi, Elena et al. "Muscle tissue changes with aging." *Current opinion in clinical nutrition and metabolic care* vol. 7,4 (2004): 405-10. doi:10.1097/01. mco.0000134362.76653.b2.

Muscle equals movement. Bones, ligaments, and tendons work together and depend upon each other to keep the car in motion. In Ancient medicine, there is a concept that explains how our bodies are both active and fixed, solid and fluid. Bones are solid to give a structure, but they're also liquid or fluid because they create bone marrow. Bone marrow is the soft portion that you see when you crack open a chicken bone, and you see the inside of the marrow, which contains white blood cells and stem cells.

Research in mice found muscles quickly produce energy and distribute it across the muscle cell through a grid-like network. The energy rate during strenuous exercise increased almost 100-fold almost instantly. To meet this demand, muscle cells contain mitochondria. These are known as "Power Plants" that convert nutrients into molecular adenosine triphosphate (ATP), which stores energy. This is known as cellular respiration or oxidative phosphorylation. They act like cellular batteries, creating an instant supply of needed energy for intense exercise and muscle strength and power.[100]

The Blue Zone Principle

Blue Zones are places in the world with the most centenarians (people who live to be 100 or longer). Within these Blue Zones, researchers have discovered that most centenarians naturally do weight-bearing exercises and live very active lives. In Sardinia, the people climb steep hills daily. In Japan, they sit on the floor, continually getting up and sitting down. Many work in the garden, chop wood, walk to get water, or work outside. So they have strong brains and strong muscles. It used to be that way all around the world, but now we live

---

[100] "Muscle Mitochondria May Form Energy Power Grid." National Institutes of Health, March 30, 2016. https://www.nih.gov/news-events/nih-research-matters/muscle-mitochondria-may-form-energy-power-grid.

sedentary lifestyles that were never intended for the optimal function of the body.

They say the strength of your legs determines the health of your brain and the length of your life. When your legs are strong, they send a signal, and blood flows through your brain. Strong legs make for strong cognitive abilities as we age. When your legs are weak, they cannot send the signal to the brain, weakening our cognitive ability as we age.[101]

Testimonial

I walked into this office looking like a zombie from pain and scarring from Shingles, but after one day of taking his supplements and ointment, I was pain-free. Shingles had left so much redness on my face, and with just one application of the ointment Scott prescribed, almost all redness went away. Scott is not only a great listener but truly God gifted with his ability to heal holistically. My whole experience was absolutely amazing as I felt like talking to a friend instead of a doctor while Scott figured out the issues and worked to create a personalized plan for my healing. Scott was so kind and listened thoroughly and, most importantly, was very empathetic. I highly recommend him for all your healing needs.
–Shelina Chandra

Miracles Are Real

For decades, I suffered a variety of bizarre symptoms ranging from dizziness to tingling extremities, food sensitivities that constantly changed,

---

[101] Yeager, Selene. "Strong Legs Tied to Enduring Brain Health." Bicycling.com, November 12, 2015. https://www.bicycling.com/training/a20049969/strong-legs-tied-to-enduring-brain-health/.

nosebleeds, a burning throat, irregular heartbeat, and skin that crawled all the time.

I was exhausted, my hair fell out, and everything hurt. I had fevers that would suddenly spike, drenching me in sweat. I had blinding headaches, liver discomfort, frequent bouts of disorientation, and blackouts.

I saw doctors, naturopaths, homeopaths, acupuncturists and integrative medicine specialists. Nobody knew what was wrong with me. After years of this insanity, I conceded that if this was how my life was going to be, I wasn't sure that I wanted it.

And then my miracle happened.

For the first time, someone understood what I was going through, and accurately diagnosed everything that was wrong with my body and the root cause of all of these issues. We started working on healing, and I'm not going to lie, there were some undeniably rough days.

Five months later, I emerged from the process, renewed. I feel 25 years younger. I feel bright, shiny, and new. I'm full of energy and optimism and fire. I feel like a giant. I am, quite literally, reborn.

What was the miracle that happened? Scott Sommer, without whom I may not be here. Gratitude always."
– Jen Wozniak

Tips

1. **Eat enough quality protein daily.** Protein builds most of the body and replaces old cells, including hair regrowth, gut and skin repair, and, of course, muscles, with each

meal for 75 to 100 g minimum. The protein requirement is based on your activity level and sex.

If you focus on getting an ideal amount of protein every day, you will reduce your calorie intake, which will help you lose weight, gain energy, and live longer.

The protein doesn't have to come from animal sources. It can be from:

- Pasture-raised organic eggs
- Wild-caught fish (especially salmon)
- Grass-fed and finished beef
- Organic chicken (eat this less often)
- Organic dairy (if you can digest it)
- Organic plant proteins
- Nuts and seeds: hemp seeds are my favorite

2. **Work out 2-3 times a week with some sort of weight-bearing exercises.** You can lift weights or dumbbells. I recommend using ankle weights while walking. You can also use exercise bands (some are better than others). We personally use a Power-Plate in our clinic for ourselves and our patients. According to the Guardian, "The Power-Plate is a machine that gives the body's muscles a high-speed workout by using vibrations to stimulate them to contract and relax. It's claimed that 10 minutes on the Power-Plate will have the same results as 60 minutes of conventional strenuous training."[102]

---

[102] "All You Need to Know about: Power-Plate." The Guardian, May 4, 2007. https://www.theguardian.com/lifeandstyle/2007/may/05/healthandwellbeing.features3.

3. **Do aerobic exercise daily for a minimum of 10-30 min daily.** Start with a 5-minute walk and slowly double it daily. Everyone has 5 minutes to exercise daily. It's important to find an exercise you can do regularly. No matter what the weather conditions are. Make sure it's simple, and you don't have to drive a distance to get there, such as a gym. We have found the best workouts are at home. Walking is the best exercise of all. Remember that aerobic exercise is great for your heart.

4. **Start jumping on a trampoline or rebounder.** I love jumping, and I've been doing it for over 25 years. Remember the story I told you about my daughter challenging me to jump rope on a trampoline? Trampolines are great for adults and children. The benefits of a rebounder or a trampoline are endless. It is my favorite exercise of all.

Story
Learning to Ride a Unicycle

My Portuguese grandmother always pushed, stretched, and taught me to grow in everything I put my hand to. She came to me one day and said, "You should ride a unicycle." I said, "I don't know how to ride a unicycle." Remember, this was before YouTube videos or the internet! She believed I could do this successfully, so I believed it, too. I practiced for hours in the garage. I fell hundreds of times, got scraped up, and scratched the car in the garage. Yet, finally, the day came when I could ride a unicycle. It was such a victorious day.

When I was ten, I started lifting weights with a bench and a barbell my dad had given me. Soon, I started jumping on trampolines, which dramatically changed my life and health. At one time, I jumped 1,000 times every morning with a jump rope while watching the sunrise and my chickens wake up in the backyard. These types of exercises have greatly helped me gain greater balance. Muscle strength, mobility, and endurance. Many people ask me how I have time to be so productive. I tell them it really comes down to how great I feel, understanding my divine purpose, and working daily on that purpose to make a difference in the world around me by sharing what the Lord has taught me.

Scan the QR Code with your Smartphone to view message about: BONES, MUSCLES AND MOVEMENT

Or follow this link: https://qrco.de/muscles_bones_movement

Afterword

A Plan and A Purpose

"Where there is no vision, the people perish."
–Prov 29:18

I found the Lord at age 9, when He gave me hope in a hopeless situation.

He taught me how to use food as medicine to heal my brain. Then, with a renewed vision for my future, I developed a passion for education. I soon realized He had also given me the gift of discernment and knowledge to heal others. This changed my life. I knew exactly what He wanted me to do, and I set out to do it.

You must find your purpose and create your plan to fulfill it. You will have joy in your heart when you have a purpose and a plan.

Finding Your Purpose

For a short time, I lost sight of my purpose. My first degree was in chemistry. I began studying chemistry and science because both were very interesting to me, but they were not my purpose or my passion. I continued on with chemical and electrical engineering. I pursued becoming an engineer but eventually realized it wasn't what I felt called to do. When I began pursuing it, I didn't ask myself, "Is this my purpose?" If I had, the answer would have been no.

After obtaining my degree in chemistry, I went to France for two years.

While I was there, I faced: a severe case of chickenpox, which became infected with oozing sores all over my body. I had to sleep with a ski cap on just to stop myself from scratching the sores on my head, and I lived in the bathtub for hours upon hours, day after day, just to stop the fevers. This went on for a month. Until I found a very good holistic doctor who came to take care of me. He gave me many different herbs and homeopathic medicine to help break my fever and alleviate the constant excruciating pain in my right leg that just wouldn't stop. It literally felt like someone was breaking my leg every hour on the mark. Before he came, nothing helped. His care ignited in me, once again, an interest in natural medicine.

Then I contracted a severe case of bronchitis from walking through Paris in the cold, brisk air. I was coughing up chunks of phlegm and on the verge of pneumonia for sure. I was again directed to a natural pharmacy (commonly found throughout France). Pharmacies in France include many natural remedies. All you must do is ask the pharmacist what to do, and they will give you what you need. In my case, the French pharmacist gave me mustard plasters for my chest to draw out the toxins and some additional remedies to help with my cough and sleep. I got through that episode of bronchitis successfully without antibiotics or any other medical intervention.

I began to think again about my future and a career in natural medicine. I had a good American friend in France whose father was a chiropractor. This was very interesting to me, so when I returned to America, I continued my education at UC Davis and decided that biochemistry was the way to meet the pre-med requirements for a medical profession. I began studying for the MCAT, the medical prerequisite for medical school. I got the books and was on my way. As I said in the introduction, I soon realized all I was learning was pharmaceuticals and surgery to become an M.D. The challenge I faced was an emptiness with this goal. For a short time, I thought I could become an M.D., and practice natural medicine. I realize now that I would have been attacked by the AMA for practicing natural medicine as an M.D. in California. I had in mind. I wanted to practice herbal medicine.

Yet soon before taking the MCAT at Davis, I read a book on traditional Chinese medicine. I was completely enthralled while reading this book for 4 to 5 hours. I was standing for the whole time and never left that spot. It talked about the electricity of the body. I suddenly realized that everything my dad had taught me was true and essential to good health (like the secret was in the soil, organic farming, food, weightlifting, bodybuilding, exercising, etc.). Still, the electricity of the body was the missing piece. Ancient medicine opened my eyes, and I was hooked. I felt God calling me to make the switch to Nutritional Science.

Knowing I needed to learn all I could about healing the body naturally; I changed my major to Nutritional Science. I continued my studies with great passion and purpose. Knowing that my goal was to use my gift of healing and discernment to help heal the world in His name. I graduated with my bachelor's from UC Davis and applied to the Pacific College of Oriental Medicine in San Diego. I then moved to San Diego, and upon graduating with my Masters of Acupuncture and Oriental Medicine (MAOM), I decided to return to Sacramento to start my own practice. I was introduced to Muscle Response Testing by a woman named Judith, who rented me the first room in downtown Sacramento to begin my practice. I was not sure about it, as it was completely foreign to me, yet soon, I realized this was the secret to customizing nutritional programs for each patient. She also introduced me to the whole food supplement company Standard Process, which has been my number one product line for healing the body naturally.

I eventually went to Florida to study Advanced Clinical Training in Kinesiology under Ulan Nutritional Systems and graduated with a certificate in Nutrition Response Testing. I also studied iridology (the study of the iris and sclerology (the white portion of the eye).

With all of these tools, I realized along the way that I was divinely directed by my education and all of the people I met along the way to help me more fully understand how to put together a system of diagnostic tools to fully understand how the body works, how we were created and how we can heal naturally. These tools sealed the deal, and from then on, my practice took off. Now, I get up every morning with a purpose and a plan, fulfilling my destiny with vibrance and passion.

As I mentioned earlier in the book, think about animals and insects. They instinctively do exactly what they were created to do every day. If they didn't, where would our world be? They each must do what they were created to do. So it is today with us. If we were all doing what we were created to do, we would live the vibrant, abundant life intended for each of us. Our lives would be full of passion and satisfaction knowing we were each fulfilling our destiny.

I pray that this book inspires you to ask yourself, "Why am I here?" What can I do to find my purpose? Always remember mine began with a prayer.

"Many are the plans in a man's heart,
but it is the Lord's purpose that prevails."
—Proverbs 19:21

I believe in inspired direction from the Lord. There is our own plan and God's plan. When something prevails, it succeeds. If you find yourself struggling with depression or anxiety about your life, perhaps you have never asked this question. The good news is that you can still change your direction and fulfill your purpose.

How will you know what that is? You will know it by the joy it gives you. God gives each of us gifts, specifically to share with the world, gifts to enable us to fulfill our purpose. Think about it. What gifts and talents do you have? What comes naturally? Go in that direction, master it, and do it for a living. If you're an artist, use it for God's Glory. Don't stay in an aimless job that keeps you from fulfilling your dreams and your God-given purpose. If you have a hobby, figure out a way to make it your own business. Find your passion, and search for ways to share it with the world. Don't accept mediocrity. Get up, get out, and make it happen!

Find your purpose and create your plan....

Be well and thrive!

Scott Sommer

"Dust off your Bible, and embrace the Ancient way of healing."
Scott Sommer, LAc

Scan the QR Code with your Smartphone to view message about Plan and Purpose

Or follow this link:
https://qrco.de/plan_purpose

Next Steps

Look for us online for further education:

- http://www.sommersholistichealth.com
  (sign up for our emails to learn about upcoming events).
- Videos on YouTube: https://www.youtube.com/
  @SommersHolisticHealth/videos
- The Podcast Channel-Life Changing Tips by Scott Sommer:
  https://open.spotify.com/show/4f0Sbk3VpAe9sn4w0GdGD1
- If you need help please call us at 916-989-0700
  or request an appointment on our website:
  https://www.sommersholistichealth.com/contact
- To order Pure Aqua Mins or Standard Process
  supplements call our office or email us at:
  frontdesk@sommersholistichealth.com

Resources

Tips on Food

I give my patients the following tips on what to eat, just to give them ideas. My wife and I practice Intermittent fasting after 3 pm, but we start our day with protein. You must get enough protein during the day to sustain muscle. We usually eat from 8 am to 3 pm. This will help with weight loss too if that is your goal. So, a great breakfast, a lighter lunch, and a light dinner, if you eat 3 meals a day.

Meal Ideas

We don't actually follow recipes; we make things up as we go, with certain key ingredients. This is the list of the things we do while working 14-hour days. If you are looking for fantastic recipes, there are many magazines and books to inspire you, such as The Whole-Body Reset, Whole 30, Engine 2, etc.

Breakfast:
We recommend high protein. If you are gluten intolerant, then you should use gluten-free options. If you are on a no-dairy regimen, eggs are a great source of protein (eggs are not a dairy product). Yogurt is dairy and causes bloating and gas for most, so we personally don't eat it. However, if you love yogurt, then eat nut yogurts like Cashew Yogurt or organic Greek yogurt. Add organic or grain-free granola, chia seeds, hemp seeds, or berries (but this can be fattening, so eat in moderation).

- **Eggs with Vegetables**: Sautéed with a small amount of avocado oil, or coconut oil, or ghee with cooked eggs separately, scrambled or over easy, etc. Sauté garlic, onions, swiss chard, red or green peppers, mushrooms, or any vegetables you prefer. Top with organic or vegan cheese (I recommend sheep cheese called Manchego or goat cheese).

- **Gluten-Free Oatmeal with Grain-Free Granola:** (organic oat groats are better than instant processed oatmeal). Add frozen blueberries or nuts. Top with a small amount of honey or maple syrup.
- **Fruit:** mandarins, bananas, berries, lemons, grapefruit, or a fruit of your choice. Start eating superfoods, such as goji berries, hemp seeds, and sachi inchi nuts.
- **Juicing:** we juice almost daily. The best juicer to buy is the Nama J2 (www.namawell.com). It's large and super easy to clean. We juice a lot of pineapple, lemon, and ginger, as well as greens, celery, apples, and carrots. Juicing will improve your complexion, and your hair, skin, and nails will become full and vibrant. If you want to lose weight, juice lemon and ginger every day.
- **Oatmeal Protein Pancakes**: Blend 2 or 3 cups of oatmeal in a blender, (use instant for pancakes). Add 1 scoop of collagen, eggs, and 1 cup of oat milk. If the batter is too thick or stiff, add more oat milk.
- Cook, add a little butter and real maple syrup.

Lunch and Dinner:
We don't usually eat after lunch. If you do eat dinner, eat early and keep it light. Fiber is important for losing weight, and with the following food choices, you should get enough fiber in your meals.

- **Grass-fed Beef, Bison, or Ground Lamb with Sauteed Vegetables and Legumes:** We mix beef, lamb, or bison with vegetables, as well as the following legumes.

Examples: kidney beans, lentils, or chickpeas. Topped with organic cheese or vegan cheese. Seasonings such as Spike® paprika, cayenne, and Redmond Real Salt® are important on both. If you eat chicken, make sure it is organic with no hormones.

- **Veggie Tacos:** organic corn tortillas warmed, with a little organic or vegan cheese, (if you prefer cheese), fill with sauteed vegetables as well as avocados, peppers, jalapeno's. You can add meat if it's organic.

- **Wild Salmon, Seabass, Wild Mahi Mahi:** these are our preferred choices when eating out or eating in. You can also use them in tacos, sauté with vegetables, or a main dish. We do not recommend shrimp, clam, or lobster as these can be very toxic to the body. Avoid all fried foods. Sides are often sweet potatoes, Brussel sprouts, salads, and organic vegetables from our garden, farmer's market, or the grocery store.

Sweet Treats and Desserts

We rarely eat desserts, but when and if we do, the following are our choices: Dark chocolate, naturally sweetened without sugar, usually sweetened with stevia, monk fruit, honey, or maple syrup.

- Frozen blueberries or any organic frozen fruit with Coco Whip (can be found at Whole Foods, Sprouts, or Nugget)
- Lily's Organic Dark Chocolate
- Melted dark chocolate with natural sweeteners
- Organic Almond Butter and melted dark chocolate also with honey
- Crepes with fruit and Coco whip

Snacks
- Organic nuts, raw and unsalted. No nuts that are coated with soybean oil or sugar. Organic trail mix, dates, and figs.
- Fruit
- Mama Chia pouches

Drinks
- 32 oz *Pressed* Juice from Costco
- GT Kombucha, Wild Tonic Organic Kombuchas with honey instead of sugar, Dr Brew Kombucha
- Mineral water
- Water with lemon or lime
- Herbal Teas
- Instant Yerba Mate sweetened with roasted stevia or unsweetened (we sell this in the clinic)
- Izzis from Costco

Eating out Locally Near Our Clinic in Rocklin, CA
- Dos Coyote: adobe salads with Mahi Mahi, Shrimp, or Salmon minimal dressing.
- Mendocino Farms: we love their Kale Salads and their menu.
- California Fish Grill: Tacos and Salads
- Vitality Bowls, Pesto Bowls and Fresh Juices
- Blaze Pizza: Cauliflower Crust, build your own
- Pottery World: Black Bean Burgers and Spinach Salads (they are only open till 3 pm).

Documentaries to Watch on Netflix:
- Forks over Knives
- H.O.P.E
- Poison
- Hungry for Change
- Fed Up
- You are What you Eat

References

The following books have been instrumental in my education, and I highly recommend them. All of these books can be found on Amazon.

Bragg, Paul C., and Patricia Bragg. *Water, the shocking truth that can save your life: The water you are drinking may look pure and safe – but is it?* Santa Barbara, Calif: Health Science, 2004.

Canfield, Jack, Mark Victor Hansen, and Les Hewitt. *The power of Focus: How to hit your business, personal and financial targets with confidence and certainty.* London: Vermilion, 2013.

Ni, Maoshing. *Secrets of longevity: Hundreds of ways to live to be 100.* San Francisco: Chronicle Books, 2006.

Gittleman, Ann Louise. *Fat Flush for Life: The year-round Super detox plan to boost your metabolism and keep the weight off permanently.* Cambridge, MA: Da Capo Life Long, 2011.

PERRINE, STEPHEN SKOLNIK, HEIDI AARP. *Whole body reset: Your weight-loss plan for a flat belly, Optimum Health & A Body You'll Love at… midlife and beyond.* S.l.: SIMON & SCHUSTER, 2024.

Bibliography

A Bitnun and R M Nosal, "Stachybotrys Chartarum (Atra) Contamination of the Indoor Environment: Health Implications," Paediatrics & child health, March 1999, https://www.ncbi.nlm.nih.gov/pmc/articles/PMC2828207/.

A., Syed S. "What to Know about Processed and Ultra-Processed Foods." News Medical, October 19, 2023. https://www.news-medical.net/health/What-to-Know-About-Processed-and-Ultra-ProcessedFoods.aspx#:~:text=Ultra%2Dprocessed%20foods%2C%20in%20contrast,instant%20soups%2C%20and%20frozen%20meals.

"About Sleep and Your Heart Health." Centers for Disease Control and Prevention. Accessed July 19, 2024. https://www.cdc.gov/heart-disease/about/sleep-and-heart-health.html?CDC_AAref_Val=https%3A%2F%2Fwww.cdc.gov%2Fbloodpressure%2Fsleep.htm.

"Acupuncture: What You Need to Know." National Center for Complementary and Integrative Health. Accessed July 19, 2024. https://www.nccih.nih.gov/health/acupuncture-what-you-need-to-know.

Aleisha Anderson, "Women's 7 Year Cycles," mke mindbody wellness, June 9, 2022, https://www.mkewellness.com/blog/2022/6/8/womens-7-year-cycles.

Alhabeeb, Habeeb et al. "Gut Hormones in Health and Obesity: The Upcoming Role of Short Chain Fatty Acids." *Nutrients* vol. 13,2 481. 31 Jan. 2021, doi:10.3390/nu13020481

"All You Need to Know About: Power-Plate." The Guardian, May 4, 2007. https://www.theguardian.com/lifeandstyle/2007/may/05/healthandwellbeing.features3.

"Allergy Facts." Asthma & Allergy Foundation of America, April 19, 2024. https://aafa.org/allergies/allergy-facts/.

Allie Wergin, RDN. "Water: Essential for Your Body." Mayo Clinic Health System, April 17, 2024. https://www.mayoclinichealthsystem.org/hometown-health/speaking-of-health/water-essential-to-your-body-video.

Anderson, Aleisha. "Women's 7 Year Cycles." mke mindbody wellness, June 9, 2022. https://www.mkewellness.com/blog/2022/6/8/womens-7-year-cycles.

Anthony, Kiara. "Lysine for Cold Sores: Treatment, Risks, and More." Healthline, March 13, 2023. https://www.healthline.com/health/lysine-for-cold-sore.

Ardeljan, Andrew D., and Razvan Hurezeanu. "Sarcopenia." National Library of Medicine, January 2024. https://www.ncbi.nlm.nih.gov/books/NBK560813/#:~:text=Sarcopenia%20is%20a%20musculoskeletal%20disease,system%20or%20impair%20physical%20activity.

"Ars Home: USDA Ars." ARS Home: USDA ARS. Accessed July 15, 2024. https://www.ars.usda.gov/.

"Bacteria." Encyclopædia Britannica, July 15, 2024. https://www.britannica.com/science/bacteria.

Baldwin, Paul. "REVEALED: How Life on Earth Began – and the Answer Is Even Crazier than You Thought." *Express UK*. August 17, 2017. https://www.express.co.uk/news/world/752936/Humans-evolved-from-MUD-says-Richard-Dawkins-bible-was-right-evolution-bible.

Barnes, Taylor. "Body Fat Percentage vs. BMI – Which Is Important?" Baylor College of Medicine. Accessed July 19, 2024. https://www.bcm.edu/news/body-fat-percentage-vs-bmi-which-is-important.

Batmanghelidj, F. *Water: For Health, for healing, for life: You're not sick, you're Thirsty!* New York: Grand Central Life & Style, 2012.

Bence, Sarah. "Grounding: Its Meaning, Benefits, and Exercises to Try." Edited by Melissa Bronstein. Verywell Health, June 14, 2023. https://www.verywellhealth.com/grounding-7494652.

Benedict Vaheems, "Companion Planting Chart and Guide for Vegetable Gardens," Almanac.com, June 5, 2024, https://www.almanac.com/companion-planting-guide-vegetables.

Biga, Lindsay M., Staci Bronson, Sierra Dawson, Amy Harwell, Robin Hopkins, Joel Kaufmann, Mike LeMaster, et al. "4.1 Types of Tissues." Anatomy Physiology, September 26, 2019. https://open.oregonstate.education/aandp/chapter/4-1-types-of-tissues/.

"Blue Zones." Bluezones.com. Accessed July 19, 2024. https://www.bluezones.com/.

Bitnun, A, and R M Nosal. "Stachybotrys Chartarum (Atra) Contamination of the Indoor Environment: Health Implications." Paediatrics & child health, March 1999. https://www.ncbi.nlm.nih. gov/pmc/articles/PMC2828207/.

Bragg, Paul C., and Patricia Bragg. *Water, the shocking truth that can save your life: The water you are drinking may look pure and safe – but is it?* Santa Barbara, Calif: Health Science, 2004.

Brain May Flush out Toxins during Sleep." National Institutes of Health, September 17, 2015. https://www.nih.gov/news-events/ news-releases/brain-may-flush-out-toxins-during-sleep.

Braun, Ashley. "What Is Heart Rate Recovery?" Edited by Jeffrey S. Lander. Verywell Health, July 20, 2023. https://www. verywellhealth.com/heart-rate-recovery-5214767.

Brody DJ, Gu Q. Antidepressant use among adults: United States, 2015–2018. NCHS Data Brief, no 377. Hyattsville, MD: National Center for Health Statistics. 2020

Circadian Rhythms." National Institute of General Medical Sciences. Accessed July 19, 2024. https://www.nigms.nih.gov/ education/fact-sheets/Pages/circadian-rhythms.aspx.

Canfield, Jack, Mark Victor Hansen, and Les Hewitt. *The power of Focus: How to hit your business, personal, and financial targets with confidence and certainty.* London: Vermilion, 2013.

Caress, Stanley M, and Anne C Steinemann. "Prevalence of Multiple Chemical Sensitivities: A Population-Based Study in the Southeastern United States." American journal of public

health, May 2004. https://www.ncbi.nlm.nih.gov/pmc/articles/
PMC1448331/.

CE;, Peden D; Reed. "Environmental and Occupational Allergies."
The Journal of allergy and clinical immunology. Accessed July 15,
2024. https://pubmed.ncbi.nlm.nih.gov/20176257/.

Center for Food Safety and Applied Nutrition. "Lead in
Cosmetics." U.S. Food and Drug Administration. Accessed July
19, 2024. https://www.fda.gov/cosmetics/potential-contaminants-
cosmetics/lead-cosmetics#:~:text=Our%20data%20show%20
that%20over,a%20maximum%20of%2010%20ppm.

Cleveland Clinic. "Health Benefits of Exercising on a Trampoline."
Cleveland Clinic, July 2, 2024. https://health.clevelandclinic.org/
trampoline-workout-benefits.

Chapman, Benjamin P, Kevin Fiscella, Ichiro Kawachi, Paul
Duberstein, and Peter Muennig. "Emotion Suppression
and Mortality Risk over a 12-Year Follow-Up." Journal of
psychosomatic research, October 2013. https://www.ncbi.nlm.nih.
gov/pmc/articles/PMC3939772/#R6.

Collier, Roger. "Swallowing the Pharmaceutical Waters." CMAJ:
Canadian Medical Association journal = journal de l'Association
medicale canadienne, February 7, 2012. https://www.ncbi.nlm.nih.
gov/pmc/articles/PMC3273502/.

Cornell University. "Clay may have been Birthplace of life on
Earth, New study suggests." ScienceDaily. www.sciencedaily.com/
releases/2013/11/131105132027.htm. (accessed July 19, 2024)

"Could Low Iron Be Making Your Mental Health Symptoms Worse?: Psychiatry: Michigan Medicine." Michigan Medicine, June 2, 2023. https://medicine.umich.edu/dept/psychiatry/news/archive/202305/could-low-iron-be-making-your-mental-health-symptoms-worse.

Davies, Dave. "Why Our Allergies Are Getting Worse -and What to Do about It." NPR, May 30, 2023. https://www.npr.org/sections/health-shots/2023/05/30/1178433166/theresa-macphail-allergic-allergies#:~:text=Estimates%20are%20that%2030%20to,U.S.%20and%20around%20the%20world.

Day, Grace. "5 Benefits to Using Bed of Nails." Beauty Bay Edited, March 25, 2022. https://www.beautybay.com/edited/bed-of-nails-benefits/.

Department of Health & Human Services. "Muscles." Better Health Channel, March 12, 2010. https://www.betterhealth.vic.gov.au/health/conditionsandtreatments/muscles.

Dewhurst, Andrea. "The Seven Year Cycle." Period Acupuncturist, December 31, 2021. https://www.theperiodacupuncturist.co.uk/post/the-seven-year-cycle.

Dr. Lana Moshkovich, "The Natural Aging Process through TCM," The Natural Aging Process through TCM: Lana Moshkovich, DACM, L.AC: Chinese Medicine, 2024, https://www.nirvananaturopathics.com/blog/the-natural-aging-process-through-tcm#:~:text=TCM%20follows%20an%208%20year,at%20the%20age%20of%208.

Dr. Liji Thomas, MD. "Irritable Bowel Syndrome (IBS) Food Triggers." News-Medical.net, September 2, 2022. https://www.news-medical.net/health/Irritable-Bowel-Syndrome-(IBS)-Food-Triggers.aspx#:~:text=Bloating%20due%20to%20bacterial%20fermentation,in%20altering%20normal%20gut%20metabolism.

Emma Loewe, "Update: The Dirty Dozen & Clean 15 Lists for 2024 Just Dropped," mindbodygreen, April 3, 2024, https://www.mindbodygreen.com/articles/ewg-dirty-dozen-and-clean-15-lists.

F. Batmanghelidj, Water: For Health, for Healing, for Life: You're Not Sick, You're Thirsty! (New York: Grand Central Life & Style, 2012).

Fish, Raymond M, and Leslie A Geddes. "Conduction of Electrical Current to and through the Human Body: A Review." Eplasty, October 12, 2009. https://www.ncbi.nlm.nih.gov/pmc/articles/PMC2763825/.

Frontera, Walter R, and Julien Ochala. "Skeletal muscle: a brief review of structure and function." *Calcified tissue international* vol. 96,3 (2015): 183-95. doi:10.1007/s00223-014-9915

George A. Parker, Tracey L. Papenfuss, in Atlas of Histology of the Juvenile Rat, 2016

Gittleman, Ann Louise. *Fat Flush for Life: The year-round Super detox plan to boost your metabolism and keep the weight off permanently.* Cambridge, MA: Da Capo Life Long, 2011.

"GMO: What Does It Mean?" Medical News Today. Accessed July 15, 2024. https://www.medicalnewstoday.com/articles/what-is-gmo.

Gora, Anna. "Is There a Link between Gut Health and Weight Loss?" LiveScience, November 3, 2022. https://www.livescience. com/gut-health-and-weight-loss&sa=D&source=docs&ust=171992 8417730223&usg=AOvVaw2yZd0f8p59d7C2L2bxs8bw.

Gropper, Sareen S. "The Role of Nutrition in Chronic Disease." *Nutrients* vol. 15,3 664. 28 Jan. 2023, doi:10.3390/nu15030664

Gut Health and Skin: How Are They Connected?" OneSkin, March 10, 2023. https://www.oneskin.co/blogs/reference-lab/ gut-health-and-skin-how-are-they-connected?u.

Harrison, Rhys, Vicki Warburton, Andrew Lux, and Denize Atan. "Blindness Caused by a Junk Food Diet." *Annals of Internal Medicine* 171, no. 11 (September 30, 2019): 859. https://doi. org/10.7326/l19-0361.

"Heartburn and Acid Reflux." NHS. Accessed July 19, 2024. https://www.nhs.uk/conditions/heartburn-and-acid-reflux/#:~:text=Causes%20of%20heartburn%20and%20 acid%20reflux&text=certain%20food%20and%20drink%20 %E2%80%93%20such,indigestion%20and%20heartburn%20 in%20pregnancy.

"Health Benefits of Dietary Fibers Vary." National Institutes of Health, June 21, 2022. https://www.nih.gov/news-events/ nih-research-matters/health-benefits-dietary-fibers-vary.

July 19, 2024. https://www.apha.org/topics-and-issues/ health-rankings.

"Healthy Habits: Antibiotic Do's and Don'ts." Centers for Disease Control and Prevention. Accessed July 15, 2024. https://www.cdc.gov/antibiotic-use/about/index.html.

"How 8 Types of Hormones Affect Your Health." Kernodle Clinic, June 25, 2020. https://www.kernodle.com/obgyn_blog/how-types-of-hormones-affect-your-health/.

Iftikhar, Noreen. "What's a Normal Blood ph and What Makes It Change?" Healthline, August 16, 2019. https://www.healthline.com/health/ph-of-blood#p-h-scale.

"Illness Causing Fish Parasites (Worms)." British Columbia: Canada, January 2013.

"IKEA Conducts Bullying Experiment on Plants – the Results Are Shocking – National." Global News, May 18, 2018. https://globalnews.ca/news/4217594/bully-a-plant-ikea/#.

Jie, Zhuye, Xinlei Yu, Yinghua Liu, Lijun Sun, Peishan Chen, Qiuxia Ding, Yuan Gao, et al. "The Baseline Gut Microbiota Directs Dieting-Induced Weight Loss Trajectories." *Gastroenterology* 160, no. 6 (January 19, 2021): 2029–42. https://doi.org/10.1053/j.gastro.2021.01.029.

Kreska, Zita et al. "Physical Vascular Therapy (BEMER) Affects Heart Rate Asymmetry in Patients with Coronary Heart Disease." *In vivo (Athens, Greece)* vol. 36,3 (2022): 1408-1415. doi:10.21873/invivo.12845

Kamrani, Payvand, Geoffrey Marston, Taflin C. Arbor, and Arif Jan. "Anatomy, Connective Tissue." StatPearls [Internet]., March 5, 2023. https://www.ncbi.nlm.nih.gov/books/NBK538534/#.

Liu, Bing-Nan, et al. "Gut microbiota in obesity." *World Journal of Gastroenterology* vol. 27,25 (2021): 3837-3850. doi:10.3748/wjg. v27.i25.3837

Loewe, Emma. "Update: The Dirty Dozen & Clean 15 Lists for 2024 Just Dropped." mindbodygreen, April 3, 2024. https://www.mindbodygreen.com/articles/ewg-dirty-dozen-and-clean-15-lists.

Lund, Mikael. "Water Experiment by Dr. Masaru Emoto." Alive Water, December 20, 2023. https://www.alivewater.ca/dr-masaru-emoto/.

Mather, Mark, and Paola Scommegna. "Fact Sheet: Aging in the United States." Population Reference Bureau. Accessed July 19, 2024. https://www.prb.org/resources/fact-sheet-aging-in-the-united-states/.

Masters, Alina et al. "Melatonin, the Hormone of Darkness: From Sleep Promotion to Ebola Treatment." *Brain disorders & therapy* vol. 4,1 (2014): 1000151. doi:10.4172/2168-975X.1000151

McGonigal, Kelly. "Five Surprising Ways Excercise Changes Your Brain." *Greater Good Magazine.* Greater Good Magazine, January 6, 2020. https://greatergood.berkeley.edu/article/item/five_surprising_ways_exercise_changes_your_brain#:~.

"Melatonin." In *Encyclopedia Britannica.* Encyclopedia Britannica. Accessed July 19, 2024. https://www.britannica.com/science/melatonin.

"Medical and Health Information | Medicalnewstoday." Medical News Today. Accessed July 19, 2024. https://www.medicalnewstoday.com/releases/163169#1.

Milcarek, Erica. "Your Feet Are Your Foundation." Active Spine & Joint, March 21, 2022. https://www.activespineandjoint.com/activesj-blog/your-feet-are-your-foundation.

Morck, T A et al. "Inhibition of food iron absorption by coffee." *The American Journal of clinical nutrition* vol. 37,3 (1983): 416-20. doi:10.1093/ajcn/37.3.416

Moshkovich, Dr. Lana. "The Natural Aging Process through TCM." The Natural Aging Process through TCM: Lana Moshkovich, DACM, L.AC: Chinese Medicine, 2024. https://www.nirvananaturopathics.com/blog/the-natural-aging-process-through-tcm#:~:text=TCM%20follows%20an%208%20year,at%20the%20age%20of%208.

"Muscle Mitochondria May Form Energy Power Grid." National Institutes of Health, March 30, 2016. https://www.nih.gov/news-events/nih-research-matters/muscle-mitochondria-may-form-energy-power-grid.

News in Health, July 2020. https://newsinhealth.nih.gov/2020/07/poor-sleep-linked-higher-blood-sugar.

Ni, Maoshing. *Secrets of longevity: Hundreds of ways to live to be 100.* San Francisco: Chronicle Books, 2006.

Nunez, Kirsten. "3 Foods (and 2 Drinks) That Can Mess with Your Hormones." Edited by Haley Mades. Real Simple, January 11, 2024. https://www.realsimple.com/worst-foods-for-hormone-health-7558543.

O'Keefe Osborn, Corinne. "Everything You Need to Know about Hormonal Imbalance." Edited by Marina Basina. Healthline, February 9, 2023. https://www.healthline.com/health/hormonal-imbalance#signs-or-symptoms.

Office of the Attorney General, Bone Health and Osteoporosis: A report of the Surgeon General. Executive summary § (2004). https://www.ncbi.nlm.nih.gov/books/NBK45513/.

"Office of Dietary Supplements – Ashwagandha: Is It Helpful for Stress, Anxiety, or Sleep?" NIH Office of Dietary Supplements. Accessed July 19, 2024. https://ods.od.nih.gov/factsheets/Ashwagandha-HealthProfessional/.

"Office of Dietary Supplements – Iodine." NIH Office of Dietary Supplements. Accessed July 19, 2024. https://ods.od.nih.gov/factsheets/Iodine-Consumer/.

"Optimum Detox Footbaths – Key Concepts, Benefits, Research, FAQ, Buyers Guide, Comparisons." Hymbas. Accessed July 19, 2024. https://www.hymbas.com/optimum-detox-footbath-key-concepts.php#Learn.

"Overview of Drinking Water Treatment Technologies." EPA. Accessed July 15, 2024. https://www.epa.gov/sdwa/overview-drinking-water-treatment-technologies.

P, Dr. Surat. "Ph in the Human Body." News Medical, October 10, 2022. https://www.news-medical.net/health/pH-in-the-Human-Body.aspx#:~:text=pH%20indicates%20the%20level%20of,is%20critical%20for%20their%20function.

"Parasitic Infection: Causes, Symptoms & Treatment."
Cleveland Clinic, 2024. https://my.clevelandclinic.org/health/
diseases/24885-parasitic-infection.

Parker, George A., and Tracey L. Papenfuss. "Chapter 10:
Immune System." Essay. In *Atlas of Histology of the Juvenile
Rat*, 293–347. Charlotte, NC: WIL Research, 2016.
https://www.sciencedirect.com/book/9780128026823/
atlas-of-histology-of-the-juvenile-rat#book-description.

Parrish, Todd B et al. "Functional magnetic resonance imaging
of real and sham acupuncture. Noninvasively measuring cortical
activation from acupuncture." *IEEE Engineering in Medicine and
Biology Magazine: the quarterly magazine of the Engineering in
Medicine & Biology Society* vol. 24,2 (2005): 35-40. doi:10.1109/
memb.2005.1411346

Pavlidi, Pavlina, et al. "Antidepressants' effects on testosterone and
estrogens: What do we know?." *European Journal of Pharmacology*
vol. 899 (2021): 173998. doi:10.1016/j.ejphar.2021.173998

"Pfas Information for Clinicians Factsheet." Centers for Disease
Control and Prevention, January 18, 2024. https://www.atsdr.cdc.
gov/pfas/resources/pfas-information-for-clinicians-factsheet.html.

Peden D; Reed CE;, "Environmental and Occupational Allergies,"
The Journal of Allergy and Clinical Immunology, accessed July 15,
2024, https://pubmed.ncbi.nlm.nih.gov/20176257/.

Per- and Polyfluoroalkyl Substances (PFAS) and Your Health."
Centers for Disease Control and Prevention, January 18, 2024.
https://www.atsdr.cdc.gov/pfas/index.html.

PERRINE, STEPHEN SKOLNIK, HEIDI AARP. *Whole body reset: Your weight-loss plan for a flat belly, Optimum Health & A Body You'll Love at... Midlife and Beyond.* S.l.: SIMON & SCHUSTER, 2024.

"Plantar Fasciitis & Foot Pain." Active Spine & Joint. Accessed July 19, 2024. https://www.activespineandjoint.com/conditions/plantar-fasciitis-foot-pain.

"Plastic Particles in Bottled Water." National Institutes of Health, January 30, 2024. https://www.nih.gov/news-events/nih-research-matters/plastic-particles-bottled-water#:~:text=T.

Raymond M Fish and Leslie A Geddes, "Conduction of Electrical Current to and through the Human Body: A Review," Eplasty, October 12, 2009, https://www.ncbi.nlm.nih.gov/pmc/articles/PMC2763825/.

Ryan, Erika, Mary Louise Kelly, and Patrick Jarenwattananon. "PFAS 'Forever Chemicals' are everywhere. Here's what you should know about them.". *All Things Considered.* NPR, June 22, 2022.

Stanley M Caress and Anne C Steinemann, "Prevalence of Multiple Chemical Sensitivities: A Population-Based Study in the Southeastern United States," American Journal of Public Pealth, May 2004, https://www.ncbi.nlm.nih.gov/pmc/articles/PMC1448331/.

Syed S. A., "What to Know about Processed and Ultra-Processed Foods," News Medical, October 19, 2023, https://www.news-medical.net/health/What-to-Know-About-Processed-and-Ultra-Processed-Foods.aspx#:~:text=Ultra%2Dprocessed.

"The Sugar That Saturates the American Diet Has a Barbaric History as the 'White Gold' That Fueled Slavery." *The New York Times Magazine*, August 14, 2019. https://www.nytimes.com/interactive/2019/08/14/magazine/sugar-slave-trade-slavery.html.

Ullah, Sana, et al. "A review of the endocrine disrupting effects of micro and nano plastic and their associated chemicals in mammals." *Frontiers in endocrinology* vol. 13 1084236. 16 Jan. 2023, doi:10.3389/fendo.2022.1084236

University of Georgia. "Low oxygen levels could drive cancer growth, research suggests." ScienceDaily. www.sciencedaily.com/releases/2012/05/120503194219.htm. (accessed July 19, 2024)

Vaheems, Benedict. "Companion Planting Chart and Guide for Vegetable Gardens." Almanac.com, June 5, 2024. https://www.almanac.com/companion-planting-guide-vegetables.

"Vibrational Products – Learn, Comparisons, Testimonials, Resources." Hymbas. Accessed July 19, 2024. https://www.hymbas.com/vibrational-machines-resources.php.

Volpi, Elena, et al. "Muscle tissue changes with aging." *Current Opinion in Clinical Nutrition and Metabolic Care* vol. 7,4 (2004): 405-10. doi:10.1097/01.mco.0000134362.76653.b2

"The Water in You: Water and the Human Body." The Water in You: Water and the Human Body | U.S. Geological Survey. Accessed July 15, 2024. https://www.usgs.gov/special-topics/water-science-school/science/water-you-water-and-human-body#:~:text=According%20to%20Mitchell%20and%20others,bones%20are%20watery%3A%2031%25.

"What Are Mitochondrial Diseases?" Cleveland Clinic. Accessed July 19, 2024. https://my.clevelandclinic.org/health/diseases/15612-mitochondrial-diseases.

"What Is Metabolic Syndrome?" National Heart Lung and Blood Institute. Accessed July 19, 2024. https://www.nhlbi.nih.gov/health/metabolic-syndrome.

Wergin, Allie. "Water: Essential for Your Body." Mayo Clinic Health System, April 17, 2024. https://www.mayoclinichealthsystem.org/hometown-health/speaking-of-health/water-essential-to-your-body-video#:~:text=Every%20day%2C%20you%20lose%20eight,a%20minimum%20of%20nine%20cups.

"What Are Mitochondrial Diseases?" Cleveland Clinic. Accessed July 19, 2024. https://my.clevelandclinic.org/health/diseases/15612-mitochondrial-diseases.

"What Is Metabolic Syndrome?" National Heart Lung and Blood Institute. Accessed July 19, 2024. https://www.nhlbi.nih.gov/health/metabolic-syndrome.

Workinger, Jayme L, Robert P Doyle, and Jonathan Bortz. "Challenges in the Diagnosis of Magnesium Status." Nutrients, September 1, 2018. https://www.ncbi.nlm.nih.gov/pmc/articles/PMC6163803/.

Yeager, Selene. "Strong Legs Tied to Enduring Brain Health." Bicycling.com, November 12, 2015. https://www.bicycling.com/training/a20049969/strong-legs-tied-to-enduring-brain-health/.

About Scott Sommer LAc

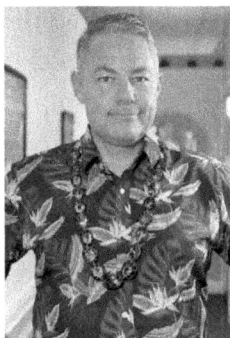

Scott Sommer LAc is a licensed Acupuncturist in Rocklin, California.

Scott started his journey in health at an early age. His father was an organic farmer, and Scott spent many days helping his dad on the farm and in the garden.

At 18 months old Scott was diagnosed with Epilepsy, and his parents did their best to help Scott battle his disease through medication and diet. At the age of nine he was told by a doctor that "if he didn't fix the epilepsy" he would never have a normal life.

Scott went home depressed and prayed, asking God to show him how to heal his own brain, promising if he would remove the disease from his own brain, he would spend the rest of his life helping others do the same.

He changed his diet and lifestyle and was declared free of epilepsy at age 15. He then went on to get a degree in Chemistry from American River College in Carmichael, CA, A Bachelor's Degree in Nutritional Science from UC Davis, a Master's in Traditional Oriental Medicine from the Pacific College of Oriental Medicine in San Diego, and then an Advanced Clinical Kinesiology Certification from Ulan Nutritional Systems, in Florida.

He began his career in 1998 in Sacramento, Ca. His clinic, **Sommer's Holistic Health** is currently in Rocklin, Ca. Scott specializes in

Holistic Family Medicine, with an emphasis on complex conditions, customized nutrition, and detox therapies.

Patients throughout the country find him in hopes of getting the help they need after exhausting all other resources. Scott's passion is helping those who have lost hope. He loves to garden, cycle, camp in his RV, and spend time with his family.

Connect with Sommer's Holistic Health
https://www.sommersholistichealth.com/
https://www.facebook.com/scottsommers
https://www.linkedin.com/in/scott-sommer-lac-85260140/
https://www.instagram.com/sommers_holistic_health/
https://www.youtube.com/@SommersHolisticHealth/videos
https://open.spotify.com/show/4f0Sbk3VpAe9sn4w0GdGD1

Sharing is Caring!

If you love what you have read, we would appreciate a review. We welcome your sharing this book with others!